T0348954

Motherdom

Motherdom

*Breaking Free from Bad Science
and Good Mother Myths*

Alex Bollen

VERSO
London • New York

For Mum
My safe haven, secure base and so much else besides

First published by Verso 2025
© Alex Bollen 2025

All rights reserved
The moral rights of the author have been asserted

1 3 5 7 9 10 8 6 4 2

Verso
UK: 6 Meard Street, London W1F 0EG
US: 207 East 32nd Street, New York, NY 10016
versobooks.com

Verso is the imprint of New Left Books

ISBN-13: 978-1-80429-753-7
ISBN-13: 978-1-80429-756-8 (US EBK)
ISBN-13: 978-1-80429-755-1 (UK EBK)

British Library Cataloguing in Publication Data
A catalogue record for this book is available from the British Library

Library of Congress Cataloging-in-Publication Data

Names: Bollen, Alex, author.
Title: Motherdom : breaking free from bad science and good mother myths /
  Alex Bollen.
Description: London ; New York : Verso, 2025. | Includes bibliographical
  references and index.
Identifiers: LCCN 2024038869 (print) | LCCN 2024038870 (ebook) | ISBN
  9781804297537 (hardback) | ISBN 9781804297568 (ebook)
Subjects: LCSH: Motherhood. | Mothers.
Classification: LCC HQ759 .B6355 2025 (print) | LCC HQ759 (ebook) | DDC
  306.874/3--dc23/eng/20241008
LC record available at https://lccn.loc.gov/2024038869
LC ebook record available at https://lccn.loc.gov/2024038870

Typeset in Sabon by Biblichor Ltd, Scotland
Printed and bound by CPI Group (UK) Ltd, Croydon CR0 4YY

Contents

Introduction

When I was pregnant, I didn't know much about what having a baby would involve, but I knew I wanted to be a good mother. After my son was born, I was dismayed to find that I felt like a bad mother, a very bad mother. I thought I was making a real mess of motherhood. My baby cried inconsolably, I struggled with breastfeeding and felt drained and bewildered. I wondered whether having a child had been a dreadful mistake. I looked to books for the answers, but this only made things worse when I read about fragile infant brains (more on this in Chapter 2).

Becoming a mother was the biggest shock of my life, and I have been trying to make sense of it ever since. I soon came to understand why early motherhood can be so difficult. Newborns need a lot of care. Broken sleep is horrible. Feeding difficulties are very common. There is often a lack of support for new mothers. Getting to grips with a new maternal identity, and all the social and psychological upheaval that entails, can be overwhelming (it can take a very long time to really feel like a mother).

Naomi Stadlen's book *What Mothers Do: Especially When It Looks Like Nothing* helped me realise that my difficulties were normal.[1] Stadlen's book draws on her weekly discussion groups with new mothers. It inspired me to become a postnatal practitioner with the National Childbirth Trust (now known as just the NCT). But I think the seeds of my interest in early motherhood were planted long before I became a mother myself. My mum was a health visitor (a public health nurse working with the families of young children) and watching her weigh babies at a baby clinic is one of my earliest memories.

I started my training as a postnatal practitioner when my second child was a few months old and have been running groups for new mothers in South West London for over a decade. Seeing women share experiences and generously support each other has been an enormous privilege. These groups have taught me a lot about early motherhood – what can help and what can make things worse.

But I continued to question why motherhood can be so challenging and guilt-ridden. There is the scrutiny and judgement that all mothers face and the vitriol around issues such as how women feed their babies or give birth. And why do women set themselves such impossibly high standards as mothers, while not appreciating all they are doing for their children? Reading Adrienne Rich's *Of Woman Born: Motherhood as Experience and Institution* was revelatory, as many others have found. Rich makes a vital distinction between the institution of motherhood – which has 'ghettoized and degraded female potentialities' – and the experience of mothering itself, which can be profoundly rich and empowering.[2]

Motherdom takes on the institution of motherhood and dismantles the Good Mother myths which underpin it. Good Mother myths are an assortment of narratives, ideologies and stereotypes. These myths are powerful and supple, with the ability to shape-shift in different times and contexts. Good Mother myths can be broad and amorphous (Good Mothers are willing to make any sacrifice for their children). They can be narrow and precise (Good Mothers gaze into their babies' eyes while they are breastfeeding) or specific but elusive (Good Mothers sculpt their children's brains). They can flatly contradict each other (Good Mothers share a bed with their babies at night; Good Mothers don't share a bed with their babies at night). They are often rooted in emotional terrain, foreclosing the possibility of negative or ambivalent feelings (Good Mothers love being with their children) or finding satisfaction outside motherhood (Good Mothers derive all their fulfilment from their children).

Good Mother myths find mothers at fault however they raise their children. As Rich memorably observed, 'the institution of motherhood finds all mothers more or less guilty of having failed their children'.[3] Good Mother myths also make mothers culpable for the ills of society. The writer Jacqueline Rose describes motherhood as 'the ultimate scapegoat for our personal and political failings, for everything that is wrong with the world, which it becomes the task – unrealisable, of course – of mothers to repair'.[4] Mother blame is deemed socially acceptable, even desirable, as mothers make convenient scapegoats for all manner of societal ills. Marginalised mothers are particularly susceptible to scrutiny and censure; vulnerable groups make easier targets.

Mothers are blamed for problems both substantial and small-scale. For instance, racial inequalities and babies' eczema are both mothers' fault according to two influential publications which appeared in 1965. The Moynihan Report, which examined the causes of Black poverty in the US, claimed that the matriarchal structure of Black families 'seriously retards the progress of the group as a whole, and imposes a crushing burden on the Negro male'.[5] In *The First Year of Life*, published in the same year, the psychoanalyst René Spitz linked specific infant ailments to maternal attitudes. So eczema is caused by 'hostility in the guise of manifest anxiety', while three-month colic is down to 'primary anxious over-permissiveness'.[6] Mother blame has perhaps never been so precise.

Perhaps the most painful element of Good Mother myths is that they draw their power from women's love and care. A key mechanism in ensuring mothers conform to Good Mother myths is dire warnings that they will damage their children. Being a Bad Mother is not just a matter of social humiliation, it means we are imperilling our children. These threats are immensely powerful, deployed to tell mothers what they can and cannot do, and shame them into compliance.

The cruellest Good Mother myths hold women responsible for the deaths of their children. The writer and medical ethicist Harriet Washington recounts how James Marion Sims, the physician infamous for conducting experiments on female slaves without anaesthesia, blamed enslaved mothers for the high death rates of their infants. He said of neonatal tetanus, which is caused by a bacterial infection: 'Whenever there are poverty, and filth, and laziness, or where the intellectual capacity is cramped, the moral and social feelings blunted, there it will be oftener found.'[7]

A more recent example was women who endured appalling maternity care at the Shrewsbury and Telford Hospital NHS Trust being made to feel responsible for the death of their babies. A review into the needless deaths and injuries of babies and mothers highlighted 'correspondence and documentation which often focussed on blaming the mothers rather than considering objectively the systems, structures and processes underpinning maternity services at the Trust'.[8]

Father blame is a much rarer phenomenon because mothers and fathers are held to very different standards. Mothers operate under a deficit model, in which any shortcomings or faults are criticised. Fathers, on the other hand, benefit from a credit model, where they are praised for anything they do. Indeed, the only common negative father stereotype is the 'deadbeat dad' who is completely absent. As the comedian Ali Wong put it, 'It takes *so little* to be considered a great dad, and it also takes *so little* to be considered a shitty mom.'[9] The writer Sara Maitland observed that her husband got 'so much praise and psychic support for doing simple things which, had I not done them, would have been considered gross inadequacy in me'.[10]

The philosopher Kate Manne's brilliantly argued book *Down Girl: The Logic of Misogyny* explains why this is the case. Women are deemed to be givers – of emotional, social, sexual, domestic and reproductive labour. We nurture, we soothe, we sympathise, we listen, we admire, we comfort, we submit ourselves. And women are not only supposed to be givers, but are required, in the words of Manne, to give in 'a loving and caring manner or enthusiastic spirit'. Men, on the other hand, are expected and entitled to be takers – of 'power, prestige, public recognition, rank, reputation, honour, "face," respect, money and other forms of wealth'.[11]

A mother/child dynamic underpins men's status as takers. The writer Siri Hustvedt observes:

> All women are expected to act on this cultural imperative: the absurd demand that I, the woman, exist only *for* you, the eternal man-child – to soothe, placate, feed, hold, admire, and adore you. And if I do not perform this part to your full satisfaction, I am a spoiled, wicked, heartless bitch – a witch.[12]

Manne explains how giver norms are enforced. Women who break them can face adverse consequences which range 'from life-threatening violence to subtle social signals of disapproval'. Women can avoid these penalties 'by being "good" by the relevant ideals or standards, if indeed any such way is open to her. Sometimes, there will not be. Double binds – and worse – are common.' As we shall see, mothers have many double binds to contend with.

Good Mother myths drive – and are driven by – expectations about how all women should behave. Women and mothers are required to be self-sacrificing, selfless and nurturing, putting others before themselves. These expectations lessen women's humanity and worth. Women are socialised from a very young age to provide caregiving labour. As the narrator of Sheila Heti's *Motherhood* observes, 'The hardest thing is actually *not* to be a mother – to refuse to be a mother to anyone.'[13]

We see motherhood norms play out in so many different ways. As a UNESCO report pointed out, most digital voice assistants, such as Alexa, use female voices, regarded as more helpful in part because of cultural perceptions of women as nurturers. These voice assistants draw upon and, in turn, reinforce beliefs that women are givers: 'It sends a signal that women are obliging, docile and eager-to-please helpers, available at the touch of a button or with a blunt voice command like "hey" or "OK".'[14]

The expectations created by Good Mother myths can be exacerbated by racist assumptions. In her essay 'Resisting Mammy Professorhood during COVID-19', the academic Jasmine Roberts-Crews writes how, like the 'Mammy' house slave figure romanticised in White imagination, she is 'expected to be unconditionally nurturing, understanding, hardworking, and mothering without an ounce of regard for my humanity or my emotional and mental health boundaries'.[15]

The Good Mother myth that children are the only path to true fulfilment devalues the lives of women who do not have children, whether through circumstance or choice (or both). As Jacqueline Rose says, 'Women who are mothers are not better or more creative than women who aren't. They have just chosen to do things differently, to live other lives.'[16] The Good Mother myth that motherhood is what women naturally desire leaves no space or understanding for women who do not want to have children. Instead, there is the implication that there is something wrong with them, they are lesser in some way. It also sharpens the pain of women who would like to have children but are not able to, for a multitude of reasons. Good Mother myths mean that women without children are subjected to scrutiny and judgement, obliging them to explain and justify their lives.

There is so much more to feminism than motherhood, and to motherhood than feminism. But they are symbiotic. The institution of motherhood underpins socially prescribed gender roles and, for marginalised women in particular, oppressive power structures. The indivisibility of womanhood from motherhood creates a double bind for all women. Women are supposed to be sexually available and attractive, but also asexual and nurturing. These are contradictory requirements and women are oppressed for both. Whether women have children or not, they should not be afflicted by Good Mother myths.

Good Mother myths derive their authority from two sources. One of these is science. I have dived deep into the scientific evidence that is used to justify prescriptions to mothers. I am a researcher with more than two decades of experience and learned my craft at the research agency MORI. We were taught that any research we published should use clear and unbiased questionnaires, be done with representative samples and have robust sample sizes. The research design should be set out in any reports or press releases and findings reported accurately. When MORI became Ipsos MORI, these standards were formalised into a process which is still known as 'Polls for Publication'. This ensures that the research design, questionnaires and write-ups are robust and transparent. During my research career, I have checked many press releases and publications written by clients who commissioned research. I've had to correct a fair few misleading headlines and unsubstantiated claims.

I naively assumed that all published research goes through a similar sort of procedure. But when I started reading studies about mothers and children, I was surprised to find – if the details were provided at all – that sample sizes were small and there was little rigour in who was selected to take part (a sample is only representative if it reflects the characteristics of the group being studied). Most of all, I was staggered by the boldness of the directives made off the back of flimsy evidence. Often, the studies cited to justify sweeping claims weren't even conducted with humans at all, but used rats or primates.

My research experience means I am well equipped to look under the bonnet of the 'evidence' base and spot the faulty wiring. Much of the 'science' which is used to chastise mothers is more akin to magical thinking – our tendency to seek spurious causal relationships to allay our anxieties – than robust scientific enquiry. Worse than that, bad science has been weaponised against women.

There is nothing new about shaky scientific claims or dire warnings from experts. I have long been fascinated by historical perspectives of bad science. I studied history at university and was struck by the bogus scientific arguments made in Victorian times to justify sexism and racism, as well as nonsensical claims that a person's character can be divined from the shape of their head. There are many good reasons to study history. For me personally, one of the most compelling is that learning about spurious theories from the past can help illuminate the present too. It is easy to mock warnings from the last century that giving babies too much attention will result in 'badly-built teeth' or that nursing and comforting a baby too much could kill them. But what will future generations make of today's claims that mothers can sculpt their children's brains by interacting with them in specific ways or politicians' calls for well-adjusted citizens whose brains have 'appropriate neural pathways'?

Bad science is one mechanism used to propagate Good Mother myths. Nature is the other and is routinely deployed to prescribe how women should both behave and feel. As the feminist Silvia Federici observes, 'If it is natural to do certain things, then all women are expected to do them and even like doing them'.[17] Sometimes science and nature are yoked together, with 'cutting-edge' science presented as revealing ancient truths.

Identifying women with nature has long been used to justify their subjugation, with social structures rooted in specific historical circumstances depicted as natural and universal.[18] It is portrayed as natural that women are maternal, nurturing and caring; women who do not behave in this way are unnatural. This means that women's work in the home and in the workplace is invisible, unappreciated and unsupported. Women are paid less and work in more precarious, undervalued jobs. Idealised notions of 'natural' mothers are an integral part of the cultural and emotional terrain of motherhood. As I explore in *Motherdom*, moral outrage against 'unnatural' mothers results in censure and harm.

I have written *Motherdom* because I am completely and utterly fed up with all the guilt-inducing garbage which is peddled about motherhood. Good Mother myths, which shame and blame women, are harmful. They can make women ill, silence their suffering and deter them from seeking help. They undermine all women, whether or not they are mothers.

I want to challenge the bad science and Good Mother myths that not only make women miserable, but also obscure what children and their parents actually need. The focus on individual relationships between mothers and children diverts our attention away from societal ills such as poverty and racism, and the wider environment of relationships and resources which children need to flourish. We must call out magical thinking on attachment and neuroscience. A secure attachment with a sensitive mother does not provide a child with miraculous protection. The notion that we can sculpt our children's brains to improve their life chances is closer to a spell than genuine scientific knowledge – and it means we're looking in the wrong place to make things better for them.

Motherdom is an angry book but also a hopeful one. We can transform our understanding and experience of motherhood, and the concept of 'motherdom' can be one of our tools. 'Condition, state, dignity, domain and realm' is what the suffix 'dom' can mean according to the *Oxford English Dictionary*. This suffix has spawned derivatives for more than a thousand years; 'motherdom' was first used in the seventeenth century.[19]

'Motherdom' should signify more than just the state of being a mother – it should also convey the dignity and power of mothers, a realm where mothers are valued and not belittled or undermined. Like freedom, 'motherdom' can express both a present reality (which may be less than satisfactory) and an ideal to strive for. And, like freedom, it can and should mean different things to different people at different times. My exploration of what 'motherdom' represents in the final chapter of this book is a beginning, not a definitive account.

I argue that 'motherdom' should denote a more generous and expansive conception of motherhood, one which values and respects the many different ways women nurture and protect their children. It should encompass a variety of mothering identities and family set-ups. The category of 'mother' should not be biologically determined. Not all mothers give birth and not all people who give birth identify as mothers. Motherdom should also embrace a broader and more constructive understanding of what children need to thrive. Instead of focusing on what mothers are doing wrong, we should ensure that parents have the resources they need to feed their children, to clothe them, to love them and to protect them from harm.

Motherdom can depose the institution of motherhood. To achieve this, we have to fiercely reject Good Mother myths. This will be immensely difficult because, as I go on to explore, Good Mother myths have great power. But we must. For children, for mothers, for everyone.

1

Good Mother Myths at Work

Some Good Mother myths are enduring – the self-sacrificing mother spans the ages – while others are particular to time and place. Good Mother myths that are historically specific are fashioned by the experts of the era and then exploited by a series of actors (including the experts themselves) for their own purposes.

In the nineteenth century, clergymen, medical men and 'pious mothers' were the key figures dispensing advice to women. Mothers were regarded, as the academic Berit Åström puts it, as important but dangerous: 'liable to destroy the child, if not closely supervised'. Mothers were instructed on their conduct, down to the tiniest detail. For instance, in a popular Victorian work, *The Management of Infancy: Physiological and Moral,* the Scottish physician Andrew Combe forbade mothers from 'endless novel-reading'.[1] During this period, moralism ruled the roost, with mothers urged to foster their children's good character through their own exemplary behaviour. 'Endless novel-reading' was apparently not regarded as setting a good example.

By the twentieth century, the emphasis had shifted to developing character through strict routines of feeding and sleeping, together with regular bowel movements. Mother blame continued though. 'At the bottom of infant mortality, high or low, is good or bad motherhood', said John Burns in London in 1906. He was president of the local government board, speaking at the first National Conference on Infant Mortality. This statement was quoted 'again and again' notes the historian Anna Davin. Infant mortality had become a matter of national concern in Britain at the beginning of the twentieth century, fuelled by anxieties about the health of the 'race' (that is, White Britons and settlers) and maintaining imperial domination.[2]

The task of tackling this was laid at the feet of mothers, who were, in the words of the academic Jane Lewis, 'held responsible for all infant deaths due to preventable causes'.[3] Similar arguments were made in the US. 'Infant mortality exists because of lack of knowledge on the part of mothers as to care of babies,' wrote Hannah Schoff, the president of the National Congress of Mothers, in 1909.[4]

Factors such as dirty milk (much milk was heavily contaminated and diarrhoea was a leading cause of death for babies in England and the US), inadequate nutrition and unsanitary housing were brushed aside.[5] Eric Pritchard, an English doctor and authority on infant care, claimed in a widely read book published in 1921: 'Infants will live and thrive in spite of poverty and bad sanitation, but they will not survive bad mothercraft.'[6]

The solution to infant mortality was, therefore, to instruct women in 'mothercraft'. 'Mothercraft' was linked not only to infant survival but also, in the words of researchers Cathy Urwin and Elaine Sharland, 'maintaining an orderly population capable of adjusting to the demands of industry or the Army'.[7] 'Mothercraft' was a neat political answer to national concerns, with mothers a convenient scapegoat. Anna Davin remarks that 'the focus on mothers provided an easy way out. It was cheaper to blame them and to organise a few classes than to expand social and medical services.'[8]

'Mothercraft' meant strict routines and behaviour. According to Pritchard, 'bad mothercraft' included feeding babies irregularly, too much and too often. An excess of care also featured in Pritchard's inventory of blame: 'they do not die because they are unloved and uncared for, they die because they are rocked and nursed and comforted too much.' In the US, the Children's

Bureau, a federal agency which was established in 1912, urged mothers to keep to rigid feeding and toileting schedules. Children needed to be taught to master their impulses and mothers were warned not to give their babies too much attention or affection.[9]

Dr Frederic Truby King, a New Zealand doctor and health reformer, was another fervent proponent of strict routines. His books became very popular in the UK, New Zealand and Australia after the First World War. He believed babies should only be fed every four hours and counselled against any feeding between the hours of 10 pm and 6 am, saying this was not 'natural and proper'. Like many who presume to tell mothers what to do, Truby King invoked nature to support his dictates. As we shall explore later in this chapter, citing 'nature' and 'instinct' are potent enforcement mechanisms for Good Mother myths.

In his popular manual *Feeding and Care of Baby*, which was first published in 1913, Truby King warned that mothers who failed to follow his instructions would ruin their babies for life:

> Nature has specially marked out the first twelve months of life as the appointed time for growing the body, and even more emphatically for growing the brain, of the human being. If the mother fritters away this one golden opportunity instead of making the most of it and doing the best possible for her baby, no after care can make up for her mistakes or neglect . . . absence of discipline and control in early life are the natural foundations of failure later on – failure through the lack of control which underlines all weakness of character, vice and criminality.

Here, 'growing the brain' in a satisfactory fashion results in good character. As we shall go on to explore, narratives around the development of the infant brain are very different now, reflecting the Good Mother myths of our era. Like other experts, Truby King weaved his admonitions about child-rearing into a wider societal narrative. He argued that mothers were responsible for the future of the British Empire, claiming 'if we lack noble mothers we lack the first element of racial success and national greatness.' He urged politicians to focus on babies and mothers 'if we wish Great Britain to be much longer great'.[10] There are echoes of this language in a 2015 report published by UK politicians, entitled *Building Great Britons,* which we shall look at in Chapter 6.

There was often a missionary impulse to expert advice. Clara Grant, a primary school teacher and settlement worker in London's East End, proudly recounted how she went about the streets of Bow snatching dummies from babies' mouths.[11] Eric Pritchard praised 'the active missionary work of whole armies of health workers' which had seen the passing of the 'old days of ignorance' where experienced mothers were seen as authorities in baby care.[12] As we shall see, the compulsion to save children from undesirable parenting has endured.

In the 1920s, the emphasis on rigid routines remained, but the justification shifted to the psychologist John Watson's behaviourism. Babies could be conditioned and good habits inculcated from birth. Experts over the years have shown varying degrees of mistrust towards mothers, but Watson is probably the most extreme example. He even contemplated getting rid of mothers altogether:

> I sometimes wish that we could live in a community of homes where each home is supplied with a well-trained nurse so that we could have the babies fed and bathed each week by a different nurse . . . Somehow I can't help wishing that it were possible to rotate the mothers occasionally too! Unless they are very sensible indeed.

Watson called mother love 'a dangerous instrument' and pronounced that mothers 'coddle' their children as a 'sex-seeking response' and because they are starved of love. Using the familiar tactic of lacing prescriptions with dire warnings, he claimed over-coddling leads to children's digestion being interfered with 'and probably their whole glandular system is deranged'.[13] Note the bogus scientific explanation being deployed here – we will see many more examples of this, past and present, in the next chapter.

Watson's and Truby King's dictates ignored the realities of women's lives, a common trait of advice givers throughout the ages. Feeding on demand allowed working-class mothers to fit baby care around their other commitments. A good mother was mainly a good worker observes the historian Ellen Ross, in her study of motherhood among the London poor in late Victorian and Edwardian times. Overcrowded housing made bed-sharing a necessity and also meant babies could be fed as soon as they cried, with less disruption for the rest of the household.[14]

Advice to schedule feeding and restrict attention was ignored by many women. In the US, the 'Plainville' community studies, undertaken in a Midwest farm community in 1939–40, found that most babies slept in their parents' beds, were breastfed on demand and were cuddled and carried when they cried. One mother explained that she raised her babies what she called the 'old way' (that is, contrary to expert advice) 'because it was easier'.[15]

At this time, expert opinion was shifting towards Plainville-style mothering. In the interwar years, the thinking of Sigmund Freud, the founder of psychoanalysis, grew in influence. Psychology was increasingly incorporated into medicine and education. The rise of fascism and the ongoing spectre of Soviet Russia fed anxieties about aggression and revolution. Expert attention turned from children's characters to their emotions, with some linking healthy emotional development to the broader national interest.[16] For instance, *The Family Book*, a collection of expert advice which was published in 1935, declared: 'The neglected toddler in everyone's way is the material which becomes the disgruntled agitator, while the happy contented child is the pillar of the State.'[17]

A profound social change which transformed attitudes towards child-rearing was the sharp decline in infant and child mortality in the West. In 1880, around 20% of babies and children died before adulthood. By 1920, the figure had dropped to 5% and it continued to decrease after that.[18] In the late nineteenth century, scientists had made the link between dirty environmental conditions and the spread of infectious diseases such as typhoid.[19] This led to public health initiatives to improve sanitation in many European and American cities, notably filtering and chlorinating water supplies and installing effective sewerage systems.[20] There were improvements in the quality of food and the safety of milk as pasteurisation became widespread. All of this resulted in dramatic reductions in infant and child deaths from infectious water- and food-borne diseases (it has been estimated that clean water and effective sewerage systems accounted for around a third of the reduction of infant deaths in Boston during this period).[21]

Mothers were not going to be let off the hook though. Instead, the 'ideology of motherhood', to use Jane Lewis's phrase, shifted from the physical to the psychological needs of the child.[22] This was fuelled by professional and commercial interests that had a stake in maternal anxiety and guilt. Historian Stephen Lassonde highlights the emergence in Europe and America in the mid-twentieth century of a corps of professionals such as academic psychologists, psychiatrists, social welfare workers, paediatricians and educators. Emphasising the need for parental vigilance, these professionals and child-rearing experts prescribed 'developmentally appropriate practices'.[23] These practices encompassed children's behaviour, physical development and what was known as 'mental hygiene'.[24]

At the same time, childhood was becoming more commercialised. For instance, the concept of the 'toddler' was invented in the 1930s, encouraged by businesses such as department stores. The historian Daniel Cook observes that 'toddler' functioned as both 'a merchandising category, an age and size range, and as new designation of the life course'.[25] Commercial and professional players with vested interests in propagating various Good

Mother myths remain powerful influences on our conceptions of motherhood.

The 1922 and 1946 editions of Mrs Sydney Frankenburg's popular manual *Common Sense in the Nursery* dealt with bad habits in very different ways. Frankenburg's expertise derived, unusually, from her own experiences as a mother of four children rather than any professional background, although she clearly kept up to date with the latest thinking on child-rearing. In the 1922 edition, she warned mothers that 'the chief point to remember about bad habits is that they should never be formed.' The shift in emphasis from children's character to emotions resulted in 'bad habits' being radically reframed in the 1946 edition: 'a bad habit is almost invariably the result of something wrong in the child's emotional life.'

Perhaps the biggest change of all was Frankenburg's treatment of masturbation. In 1922, she warned that '*undesirable handling*' (italics in the original) was the most dangerous habit of all in young children, risking both moral and physical peril. In contrast, the 1946 edition has a matter-of-fact discussion about masturbation (now named) and reassurance that it does not result in 'evil effects'. Frankenburg kept her foot in both the Freudian and behaviourism camps though. In 1946, she was still quoting Truby King and Pritchard and advocating 'absolute regularity' in feeding schedules, no feeding at night and bowel movements 'at a fixed time daily'. A sentence that appeared in the 1946 edition illustrates how she blended advice from two different eras: 'Be careful to show your love – without being emotional of course.'[26]

It was the book *Babies are Human Beings*, published in 1938 in the US and 1939 in the UK, which marked a clear break with previous advice. It became a bestseller in the US within a year of publication and heavily influenced later experts, most notably Dr Spock, who we shall come to shortly. Written by the paediatrician Anderson Aldrich and his wife Mary Aldrich, it was inspired by psychoanalytic thinking. It advocated a 'deep-seated recognition of the importance of individual differences' and told parents to 'adjust our habit-training to his individual rhythm'. In the interests of 'mental hygiene', parents were urged 'to give a baby all the warmth, comfort and cuddling that he seems to need'.[27] Cathy Urwin and Elaine Sharland note that in the Aldrichs' book, cuddling 'became not only acceptable but essential'.[28]

By the 1940s, Freudian thinking reigned supreme. Mothers were now held responsible for their children's emotional adjustment and personality development. Edicts to restrict attention and stick to strict schedules were replaced by advice advocating affectionate parenting. As the historian Janet Golden points out, there was no acknowledgement from psychologists or physicians in America that they were endorsing practices common among generations of urban immigrants, Native Americans and rural farm families.[29]

However, previous injunctions were still in circulation. In her qualitative research with different generations of Oxfordshire mothers, the historian Angela Davis found that Truby King's edicts were still influencing mothers in the 1940s, 1950s and even early 1960s.[30] Having to navigate conflicting currents of advice is one of the double binds of motherhood.

The most influential expert in the post–Second World War era was the paediatrician Dr Benjamin Spock. He famously told parents, 'Trust yourself. You know more than you think you do.' His book *The Common Sense Book of Baby and Child Care* (later called just *Baby & Child Care*) was first published in 1946. By 1998, the year of Spock's death at the age of 94, it had sold over 50 million copies and been translated into 39 languages.[31]

Spock was from an affluent New England family (he won a gold medal for rowing at the 1924 Olympics in a Yale University boat). Similar to John Bowlby, the father of attachment theory who we will encounter in Chapter 5, his childhood was cold and austere. Spock, again like Bowlby, was heavily influenced by Sigmund Freud, although he didn't mention Freud by name until the 1968 edition of his manual. He feared that Freud was too controversial for an American audience, having heard people make comments such as 'he sees everything as sexual.'[32] Rather than strict feeding schedules, Spock advised mothers to be 'flexible and adjust to the baby's needs and happiness'. He warned that trying to make an 'irregular baby' have regular bowel movements was unrealistic and ran the risk of 'upsetting the baby emotionally'.

Like Bowlby, Spock's views were strongly shaped by contemporary gender ideology; a mother's place was in the home. In a section on working mothers (which appears in a chapter called, tellingly, 'Special Problems') he wrote:

> Useful, well-adjusted citizens are the most valuable possessions a country has, and good mother care during early childhood is the surest way to provide them. It doesn't make sense to let mothers go to work making dresses in factories or tapping typewriters in offices, and have them pay other people to do a poorer job of bringing up their children.[33]

However, unlike Bowlby, Spock's views evolved. He took on board the forceful criticisms made by feminists such as Gloria Steinem in the 1970s. He became involved in progressive politics and was sentenced to jail in 1968 on charges of conspiracy to aid resistance to the Vietnam War draft. He even ran for president of the US in 1972 as the People's Party nominee.[34] In the 1976 edition of *Baby & Child Care*, Spock acknowledged feminist thinking. Spock later said that it took him 'three years of discussions with many patient women before I fully understood the nature of my sexism'.[35] In the updated *Baby & Child Care*, he argued that both parents have an equal right to a career and equal obligation to share in the care of their child.[36] However, the focus on the emotional needs of children remained the same.

Although strict routines were out of fashion by the 1940s, calamitous warnings that women could ruin their children endured. Mothers were variously blamed for juvenile delinquency, alcoholism and homosexuality (which at the time was generally regarded as an illness), and held responsible for producing rapists, communists and men who were unfit for military service.[37] In their best-selling 1947 book, *Modern Women: The Lost Sex*, the sociologist Ferdinand Lundberg and psychiatrist Marynia F. Farnham drew heavily on Freudian thinking to argue that mothers were messing their children up – and ruining society in the process. They wrote, 'The spawning ground of most neurosis in Western civilisation is the home. The basis for it is laid in childhood . . . the principal agent in laying the groundwork for it is the mother.'[38]

The success of *Modern Women: The Lost Sex* was part of a backlash against the expansion of women's employment during the Second World War.[39] It sought to provide scientific justification for confining women's time and energies to the home. The arguments made were often absurd. For instance, the book spends ten pages attempting to prove that feminist philosopher Mary Wollstonecraft 'was afflicted with a severe case of "penis-envy"'. Wollstonecraft was, we are informed, 'an extreme neurotic of a compulsive type' and 'out of her illness arose the ideology of feminism'.

Lundberg and Farnham catalogued four different ways in which women damaged their children: being rejecting, being overprotective, being dominating and being over-affectionate. It was claimed that being over-affectionate caused the most 'damage' with sons 'whom she often converts into "sissies" – that is, into passive-feminine or passive-homosexual males'.[40]

Mid-century psychology effectively left women walking a tightrope, where they needed to avoid being overinvolved or underinvolved with their children.[41] Adrienne Rich wrote of her realisation of this after the birth of her first son, 'Soon I would begin to understand the full weight and burden of maternal guilt, that daily, nightly, hourly, *Am I doing what is right? Am I doing enough? Am I doing too much?*'[42]

The Intensification of Motherhood

Although the tightrope was challenging to traverse, it at least offered mothers a pathway of sorts. The 1977 book *Fathers, Mothers, and Others*, which evolved from a literature review commissioned by the UK government, suggests charting a course between doing both too much and too little: 'The child-centred parent who is responsive to every word, facial expression, cry or step of the child is at one extreme – and the neglectful, indifferent, perhaps abusive parent at the other.' The authors warned that parents need to avoid martyrdom and children have to 'come to terms with the idea that the world is not organised to gratify him/her alone'.[43]

It is very hard to imagine something like that being written today. Good mothering now requires doing whatever might enhance children's physical, intellectual and emotional development. The phrase 'it's never too early to start . . .' routinely appears in advice. The emphasis is on doing *more* and *sooner*. And the pressure starts before babies are even born. For instance, in the 'red book', the personal child health record provided by the National Health Service (NHS), an insert written by UNICEF UK declares, 'The more you take time out to connect with your unborn baby the more you help her brain development. You can feel proud that you are giving your baby the best start in life.'[44]

There is absolutely no evidence for this assertion. And logically it is nonsense, a point I shall make again because it is so important to call this drivel out. There is a ceiling to any form of development, it cannot be infinite.

Ludicrous though it is, this advice reflects the Good Mother myths which pervade our culture; there is no ceiling on what we expect mothers to do for their children. We are now in the era of 'intensive mothering', a term coined in 1998 by the sociologist Sharon Hays. She defines intensive mothering as 'child-centred, expert-guided, emotionally absorbing, labour-intensive, and financially expensive'.[45]

The experts tell us what is best, or 'optimal', a word peppered throughout current advice, doubtless because it carries a veneer of scientific authority. For instance, in a book by the child psychologist and psychotherapist Margot Sunderland, which we shall look at in more detail in Chapter 6, there is an entire chapter on the 'best' relationship with your child, which promises 'a whole host of practical and fun-packed ideas – all backed by brain science'. Sunderland advises that parents who want the 'best' relationships should carry on massaging their child beyond babyhood, while the 'best' way to communicate is, apparently, baby signing.[46]

The need to achieve the 'best' is now a pervasive Good Mother myth, a central plank of intensive mothering. The requirement for parents (which in reality means mothers) to be the 'best' is seen in the Graded Care Profile tool used in the UK by child protection workers to identify neglect. Grade 1 is judged to be the 'best' care and Grade 5 the 'worst'. To achieve a Grade 1, parents have to be 'child first'. If your child is merely your priority, you get a Grade 2, which is only 'adequate' care.[47] A version of the manual published by a local authority sets out what this means in practice. These are examples of providing the best (Grade 1) care: starting more interactions with the child than the child starts with the parent; praising the child without being asked; and responding at the time of the child's signals or even before in anticipation. Care is merely 'adequate' if interactions are started with equal frequency, parents talk fondly about the child when asked instead of spontaneously and mostly respond to the child's signals straight away.[48] This is the codification of intensive mothering. Could *anyone* realistically achieve the 'best' grade?

And why should we expect parents to aspire to these standards? The requirement to provide the 'best' allows no room for diversity (there is the best and then everything else) or for a woman's own judgement about her individual family (the experts like Sutherland tell us what is best) or her preferences or her circumstances or her culture (she may not have the time or money for baby signing classes, she may feel it is inappropriate to lavish praise on children). It also goes against the vast expanse of human history. If there really is one 'best' way to do things, how have human beings managed to survive and thrive in so many different contexts?

The rise of intensive mothering needs to be seen in the context of significant economic and social changes in the West since the 1970s. The male-breadwinner and female-housewife model has been eroded. Maternal employment has steadily risen and rates of divorce have increased. Traditionally male sectors such as manufacturing have declined and jobs have become less secure. Women have entered traditionally male professions such as law, medicine and accountancy.[49]

Intensive mothering is a reaction to the (limited) economic and social gains women have made because, as Sharon Hays points out, it helps reproduce gender inequalities. The difference is that women are now confined to the nursery rather than the kitchen. The journalist Amy Senior notes the shift in terminology from the 'housewife' to 'stay-at-home mom', with the change in emphasis from keeping an immaculate house to being a perfect mother. In parallel, there is now the same differentiation between baby toys (problem solving versus encouraging imaginary play) as there was between cleaning products in the 1950s. The expectation in both cases is that women will eagerly master these nuances.[50]

Rising inequality is also an important factor at play. The economists Matthias Doepke and Fabrizio Zilibotti have linked the growth in intensive parenting to this, along with higher education becoming 'an essential precondition for economic and social success'. Parenting in more egalitarian countries such as Sweden tends to be more laid back than in countries like the US and UK: 'when economic inequality is low or when there are plentiful opportunities for children doing "just fine" to enjoy a comfortable middle-class life, the stakes in parenting are also lower, and parents can afford to be more relaxed.'[51]

The ideology of intensive mothering excuses and explains economic and racial inequalities by holding mothers responsible for their children's outcomes. We have seen how mothercraft was once touted as the solution to disease, contamination and insanitary living conditions. Now intensive mothering is deployed as both the reason for and solution to enormous disparities in opportunities and resources. In the era of neoliberalism, where individual responsibility holds sway, social services and welfare safety nets have been weakened. Many of the services once provided by government, such as recreation, health, culture and carework, have been 'downloaded to mothers', to quote Andrea O'Reilly, a pioneer of scholarship on motherhood.[52]

The growth of risk culture is another powerful motor in the intensification of motherhood. The academic Joan Wolf argues that we are in an era of 'Total Motherhood', a moral code which involves not just 'optimisation' from the womb but also reducing any perceived risks to the child, regardless of how small these might be.[53]

A striking example of how much attitudes have changed comes from a tremendous piece of work from the sociologists Rosalind Edwards and Val Gillies. They revisited the fieldnotes and accounts of interviewers from two classic 1960s studies among English working-class families. The researchers made very judgemental remarks about the study participants' intelligence and appearance; the mothers were variously described as 'greasy, spotty, fat, simple, spineless and lacking sex appeal'. However, no comment at all was passed upon young children being regularly left home alone, or babies and toddlers being routinely cared for by very young siblings. Edwards and Gillies remark that 'widely accepted practices and values from the 1960s . . . would today be viewed at best in terms of benign neglect and at worst as child abuse'.[54]

Framing anything in terms of 'risk' intensifies the stakes. Risk is a statistical term which signifies the likelihood of something happening, but it is laden with negative associations of danger and peril. Why would any mother want to put her child in harm's way? To allow any sort of risk is presented as negligent and dangerous, although the reality is that it is impossible to lead a life free of risk. It is another unattainable Good Mother myth.

Risk and morality are interwoven. The writer Sarah Menkedick has considered how anthropologist Mary Douglas's observation that risk prescribes social values applies to motherhood:

> These values include the sanctity of the child, the perfectibility of the child, the sacrificial nature of motherhood, and the responsibility of the individual for maintaining his or her own 'wellness'. Risk is a way of policing and reinforcing these values. We chart the lines of social purity and transgression with the chalk of risk, and when disaster strikes, we blame the individual for not hewing closely enough to them.[55]

The chalk lines of risk encompass pregnancy, and the need for vigilance starts before a baby is even conceived. 'Drinking alcohol BEFORE pregnancy can alter your baby's face, study finds' was the headline of a piece on Netmums, a UK parenting website.[56] This particular study used artificial intelligence to analyse three-dimensional images of children taken at the ages of nine and thirteen. Images were broken down into 200 facial traits and, at the age of nine, three (just three!) of these traits were different among mothers who reported drinking before pregnancy compared with mothers who did not. It is hard to see how these miniscule differences constitute changing a child's face. Nevertheless, the study concludes that women 'should quit alcohol consumption several months before conception'.[57]

This is a good example of using shaky science to instruct women (more on this in the next chapter). Telling women to stop drinking before conception is more about morality than avoiding any actual risk. We can see how morality shapes attitudes towards risk when we think about cars. Motor vehicle accidents are a leading cause of death among under-fives in the US, but no one campaigns to ban cars or suggests that only bad mothers and fathers put their children in cars.[58]

One of the reasons why risk culture is so persuasive is that any verdict on how children turn out is postponed far into the future (if ever possible at all). Intensive mothering is a way to hedge against these risks. Simon Dein, an anthropologist and psychiatrist, argues that risk, like witchcraft and magic in other societies, 'plays a central role in making the future more predictable and manageable'. Identifying and tackling risks attempts, Dein observes, to 'diminish uncertainty'.[59] But, as Menkedick puts it, 'the second one concern has been "controlled" another rears its head and whispers, *look out*, and like whack-a-mole it has to be smacked down, and then ten more pop up.'

Anxiety levels are ramped up as even the smallest decisions about child-rearing are framed as having long-lasting consequences. But mothers are also instructed to relax, 'to mime the serenity of madonnas', as Adrienne Rich memorably put it, and enjoy their children.[60] The requirement to relax against a backdrop of the stakes being presented as enormously high is one of the double binds of motherhood.

The Unequal Burden of Intensive Mothering

The Good Mother myth of intensive mothering sets up all mothers to fail, but women who are not White, middle class, heterosexual and able-bodied are especially vulnerable to censure. In her essay 'The Impossibility of the Good Black Mother', the writer T. F. Charlton observes:

> As mothers, we belong to a global sorority of women labouring under expectations that our parenting be open to any and all interrogation. But as with any oppression, we don't share this burden evenly or identically . . . The Good Mother is married to the father of her children, nurturing to the point of self-abnegation,

a model of middle-class domesticity . . . The images projected on me as I walk my neighbourhood streets are not the Good Mother. No, they are of the Black welfare queen, the baby mama, of women maligned and demonised as everything should not be, foil and shadow to the Good (White) Mother.[61]

The social theorist Patricia Hill Collins describes how assorted 'controlling images' – 'stereotypical mammies, matriarchs, welfare recipients, and hot mommas' – are used to justify Black women's oppression in the US. Double binds are busy at work here. Black women who work are the 'Black matriarchs' who the Moynihan Report conjured up to reproach for racial inequalities. But Black mothers who do not work are portrayed as 'welfare queens' who are to blame for their own poverty and their children's constrained life chances.

These controlling images keep the gaze of judgement firmly focused on Black mothers, instead of wider economic and political inequalities. As Collins observes, 'portraying African-American women as matriarchs allows White men and women to blame Black women for their children's failures in school and with the law, as well as Black children's subsequent poverty.' Simultaneously, the welfare mother stereotype 'shifts the angle of vision away from structural sources of poverty and blames the victims themselves'.[62]

Women lacking the resources or circumstances to enact intensive mothering carry a heavy burden as they are held to standards which are even more unrealistic. In their qualitative research among low-income Black single mothers in the US, the sociologists Sinikka Elliott, Rachel Powell and Joslyn Brenton conclude that intensive mothering 'increases their burdens, stresses, and hardships even while providing a convenient explanation for these very difficulties: *mothers* are to blame'. The women wanted to protect and do their best for their children. This required 'fending off the dangers, indignities, and vagaries of poverty, racism, and sexism'.[63]

Protecting children from dangers and indignities is an example of what Patricia Hill Collins has described as 'motherwork' – 'women's unpaid and paid reproductive labor within families, communities, kin networks, and informal and formal local economies'. For Black mothers, motherwork involves ensuring their children's physical survival (which Collins notes is 'assumed' for White children) and 'negotiating the complicated relationship of preparing children to fit into, yet resist, systems of racial domination'.[64]

This motherwork is agonising and goes unrecognised. The legal scholar and sociologist Dorothy Roberts wrote in a 1993 essay:

> Most white mothers do not know the pain of raising Black children in a racist society. It is impossible to explain the depth of sorrow felt at the moment a mother realizes she birthed her precious brown baby into a society that regards her child as just another unwanted Black charge. Black mothers must bear the incredible task of guarding their children's identity against innumerable messages that brand them as less than human.[65]

Motherwork for women living in poverty can also be unseen and unappreciated. Mothers on meagre incomes must undertake complex labour to meet their children's needs. The sociologist Jennifer Randles has coined the term 'inventive mothering' to convey the resourcefulness and ingenuity employed by women. In her qualitative research among Californian mothers experiencing 'diaper need' (that is, lacking sufficient diapers to keep a child dry, comfortable and healthy), she found that 'extensive physical, cognitive, and emotional labor' is required. Women had to meticulously manage their diaper supplies; most knew exactly how many diapers they had and how long the diapers would last. Some had gone without food to save diaper money, and many had avoided leaving home. Most had experienced running out of diapers at some point and had improvised with household materials, such as paper towels, dish cloths, pillowcases and T-shirts. Ensuring their babies had diapers was an act of care, love and pride.

Unmothering: The Ultimate Sanction

Diaper work is also an undertaking of vigilance and defence. Latina and Black mothers taking part in the study were afraid of losing custody if their children wore soggy or smelly diapers, fears that were grounded in reality. Several of the mothers (all Black) lost custody of older children to the child welfare system or had grown up in it themselves.[66]

Black feminist scholars have identified 'unmothering' as central to Black women's maternal experiences in the United States. The institution of slavery was built around, in the words of Black feminist theorist Jennifer C. Nash, 'the literal violent tearing apart of families'.[67] Unmothering, the removal of children and denial of a woman's motherhood, continues to haunt Black mothers. Black women are more likely to have their newborn placed in someone else's care. Black children are more likely to be taken into foster care than children of other races and are less likely to be reunited with their mothers.[68]

Unmothering plays out in different ways across different societies but is generally more of an acute threat for women from marginalised groups. A blind woman who took part in Angela Frederick's qualitative research among US and Canadian mothers with physical and sensory disabilities was frightened of her baby being taken away. She had heard of two recent cases of newborns of blind parents being placed into state custody solely because of the parents' disabilities: 'It's just terrifying. Even like with the breastfeeding, I just felt like, "Oh God, I gotta do this perfect the first time or they're gonna take my kid away."'[69]

The academic Margaret Gibson explains how queer mothers have to bring their children up under the shadow of unmothering:

We are asked, again and again, to assert a conviction that our children can, and will, be 'okay,' which usually means, 'absolutely indistinguishable from kids of idealized heterosexual, middle-class, white, able-bodied, etc. etc. parents'. The stakes are high. These defences of our children and our parenting capacities have been made under the fear of losing custody of our children or of losing the possibility of having children in the first place.[70]

'Married' isn't in Gibson's list of desirable attributes, but at one time it was a prerequisite for being a Good Mother. The sanction of unmothering was applied to women who had babies out of wedlock. From the 1940s to the 1970s, hundreds of thousands of unmarried women in the US, Canada, the UK, Australia, New Zealand and Ireland were coerced into giving their babies up for adoption.[71]

In the US, this pressure was only applied to White women. The historian Rickie Solinger recounts how unmarried Black mothers were regarded as 'innately biologically flawed by hypersexuality'. It was thought they should be punished by being made to keep their babies but excluded from welfare assistance. These beliefs were also used to justify sterilising Black girls and women. The pregnancies of unwed White women, on the other hand, were attributed to mental illness, which was deemed to be curable. White children born out of wedlock were no longer regarded, in the words of Solinger, as 'a flawed by-product of innate immorality and low intelligence'. They were therefore now suitable for adoption by a 'deserving' family. This course of action also rehabilitated the child's mother who was, after losing her baby, able to achieve motherhood the appropriate way, through marriage.[72]

Parliamentary inquiries in Australia and Canada have examined how forced adoption happened and its devastating impact on women and the children removed from them.[73] Churches, governments and charities, often operating through maternity homes, colluded to remove newborn babies from their mothers. In Canada, quotas were even set for the number of babies to be surrendered to the adoption system. In some cases, consent was given under duress, or not at all. Babies were simply taken away. One Australian woman recalled: 'I was devastated when she was wrenched from my arms. No one spoke to me as my baby vanished from my sight.' Some women never saw their babies and were falsely told they had died.

Where women did consent to adoption, they were generally given no other options and pressurised by maternity homes, health professionals and their parents. One Australian woman said 'We were subjected to intense propaganda, aimed at having us relinquish our babies. The most common line being: if we *really* loved our babies we would give them away, to a proper two parent family.' These women were disbarred from motherhood simply because they were not married. One recounted, 'I was told . . . what an evil girl I was, that I could never be a proper mother to my baby and the Sisters of St Joseph would help me give my baby to a real mother.'

In America, Australia, Canada and New Zealand, Indigenous children were also systematically removed from their families during this period, and for many years before.[74] Children were not allowed to use their language, their names were changed and some were told their parents did not want them or were dead. Many endured awful cruelty and hardship in their new homes. In Australia, this policy was known as 'assimilation', with a government minister explaining in 1953 that the aim was that 'in the course of time, it is expected that all persons of aboriginal blood or mixed blood in Australia will live like other white Australians do'.[75] In his 1985 review of removals of Indigenous Canadian children from their parents, Judge Kimelman concluded that 'cultural genocide has been taking place in a systematic, routine manner'. It was not only their mothers who were deemed unworthy of these children, but also their families, communities and culture. Kimelman was particularly critical of the failure of social workers to understand or respect communal patterns of care. He wrote 'life for a child . . . is one of safety, love, adventure, and freedom. A child feels, and is, welcome in any home and may join any family for a meal.'[76]

Unmothering continues to impact some ethnic groups more than others. As we have seen, Black children in the US are more likely to be removed from their families. In Canada, Australia and New Zealand, disproportionate numbers of Indigenous children are taken into care.[77] In the UK, levels of intervention vary according to both ethnicity and deprivation in the local area (assessed through indicators such as income, employment, education and health). In neighbourhoods of high deprivation, Black Caribbean children are over twenty times more likely than Asian Indian children to be in care. White British children, on average, have higher rates of intervention than children from other ethnic groups in poorer neighbourhoods and lower rates in more affluent neighbourhoods.[78]

Poverty is a significant dynamic in the removal of children from their families. In the UK, the more deprived an area a child is living in, the higher their likelihood of being taken into care. Children living in the most deprived 10% of neighbourhoods are more than ten times as likely as children in the least deprived 10% to be in care or on child protection plans. More than half (55%) of children in care or on protection plans live in the most deprived 20% of neighbourhoods.[79] One study found that a one percentage point increase in child poverty in England was associated with an extra five children per 100,000 children being taken into care. While correlation is not causation, as we shall go on to explore in the next chapter, the researchers contend that other evidence suggests a causal effect between family income and entering child protection systems.[80]

However, poverty is 'curiously invisible' in child welfare policy and practice according to the academics Brid Featherstone, Anna Gupta, Kate Morris and Sue White.[81] For instance, in the Graded Care Profile manual referred to earlier, families are assessed on the quality and quantity of nutrition provided and the maintenance of, and décor and facilities in, the home (décor is Grade 1 if it is 'excellent, child's taste specially considered').[82] There is no acknowledgement of the difficulties parents on low incomes living in substandard housing may face in meeting these criteria. In her book *Torn Apart*, Dorothy Roberts points out that many indicators used by agencies to evaluate risks for maltreatment, such as lack of food and insecure housing, are actually conditions of poverty.

Dorothy Roberts characterises the child welfare system in the US as a 'family-policing system'. She describes it as a form of 'benevolent terror' which tears families apart, particularly Black and Indigenous families. She estimates that ten times as much funding is spent on separating children from their parents than on keeping families together. As in the UK, children's welfare is addressed through fixing perceived parenting deficits. Failing to co-operate with these requirements risks children being taken away. Roberts relates the experiences of the Black mothers she got to know:

> The prescribed solutions to their problems were a far cry from material things they said they needed, such as cash, affordable housing, furniture, food, clothing, education, and child care. Often, the requirements had nothing to do with their needs at all – like ordering them to attend anger management classes or treatment for drug addiction when they didn't have a problem with anger or drugs. The mothers regarded them more as assignments they had to complete to get their children back than as real assistance to their families . . . In fact, the dizzying catalogue of burdensome and conflicting obligations made it harder for the mothers to take care of their children or prepare to reunite with them.[83]

Unmothering is fuelled by mother blame. The threat of it puts a heavy burden of responsibility on women bringing up children in difficult circumstances to protect them from poverty, poor housing and violent partners. The focus on mothers in child protection can also mean discounting fathers and other family members; one paper argued that the child welfare system manufactures 'ghost fathers' who are invisible, whether they are risks or strengths for their children.[84]

Some women are not given any opportunity to mother at all. Most US states remove babies born in prison from their mothers.[85] In England, there has been a sharp rise in the number of children born into care and taken away from their mothers at birth; the rate almost doubled over a ten-year period. While there is a clear relationship between deprivation in the local area and the number of babies being taken into care at birth, there are some wide variations between local authorities. Most starkly, one baby in every forty-six born in Blackpool in 2017–18 was taken into care at birth.[86]

One reason for the rise in newborns being removed is that years of austerity in the UK have hollowed out services and support for vulnerable new mothers. A qualitative study among social workers in England and Wales found they were left with few options because of housing shortages, insufficient support for addiction or domestic abuse provision and a lack of mother and baby placements. One social worker said, 'when we are writing our assessments in terms of identified risk, a lot of the times we have to say removal at birth because there are no facilities'.[87]

Another factor is the influence of an early intervention philosophy, underpinned by neuroscience and attachment theory, which stresses the critical importance of the early years. A UK review for professionals involved in care proceedings states:

Abuse and neglect in infancy and early childhood will have a significant impact on the child's neurobiological development and on their capacity to form attachments. Unless effective action is taken, such experiences can have a long-term, negative impact on all areas of physiological, cognitive, social, behavioural and emotional development.[88]

This claim is based on shaky foundations, as we shall go on to explore in later chapters, but it has helped to fuel an increase in the number of child protection cases in the UK. More cases now relate to children aged zero to four and to emotional abuse, while numbers have declined for both physical and sexual abuse cases.[89]

Women under threat of having their babies removed at birth are put in the unbearable position of either missing out on precious time with their baby by going to court or staying with the baby and risking reproach for not attending legal proceedings on their baby's future. Social services' assessments during pregnancy require evidence that prospective parents are investing financially and emotionally in their baby, but this means that mothers who have their baby removed have to return alone to a home full of baby items. One woman said, 'All his stuff was upstairs. I couldn't even bear to look at it. It was locked in the spare room and that was it . . . I was alone. I was on my own. Nobody to speak to. Nobody to comfort me. Nobody.' Another woman took an overdose when she returned home alone 'because I didn't want to be alive without my baby'.[90]

Removing a child from their family is a grave act which can result in enduring sorrow, anguish and trauma. This is clear from the testimony of witnesses to the Australian inquiry into the forced adoption of babies of unmarried mothers. One woman said, 'I have suffered a lifetime of grief and pain, crying every day for my son, and the loss of him.' An adoptee stated that 'being brought up by strangers left me with identity confusion, a sense of not fitting, of being a fraud, an inability to maintain relationships and a belief that I was unlovable.'[91] In the 1997 inquiry into the removal of Aboriginal children from their families, one woman poignantly recalled the one and only encounter she had with her mother, who died two years later:

When I first met my mother – when I was 14 – she wasn't what they said she was. They made her sound like she was stupid, you know, they made her sound so bad. And when I saw her she was so beautiful. Mum said, 'My baby's been crying' and she walked into the room and she stood there . . . I walked into my mother and we hugged and this hot, hot rush just from the tip of my toes up to my head filled every part of my body – so hot. That was my first feeling of love and it only could come from my mum. I was so happy and that was the last time I got to see her.[92]

These inquiries took place to investigate and acknowledge the harm caused by forced removals. However, the consequences of unmothering often remain hidden from view because the women and children experiencing the fallout are marginalised and powerless. When we do hear mothers' voices, their pain rings out. In a qualitative study among Canadian women, mothers recounted how the removal of their children led to a profound sense of loss. The women no longer felt like mothers. One said:

I don't feel like my kid's mother any more. I really don't . . . It's hard to wake up day in and day out in the same house with all their toys and every time I turn round there's something of theirs there and there's not them there . . . Everyday, you know, it takes a piece of you away.[93]

Children must be protected from violence, abuse and neglect. And there are, of course, cases where removing a baby or child from their mother and family is the only way to do this. But the current deficit model of mothering, unmoored from economic, social and cultural factors and fortified by racism, classism, ableism and homophobia, is a very unforgiving one. How far can we justify the pain and trauma caused when children are taken from their families? As Sue White, a professor of social work, said to the *Guardian* journalist Zoe Williams: 'It's only when the children who've been removed grow up, and ask, "But did anybody try to help my mum?" '[94] This is a crucial issue, and one we shall return to in the final chapter of this book.

While unmothering is a much greater risk for marginalised and vulnerable women, it is the ultimate sanction for all mothers. It is a key mechanism in enforcing Good Mother norms. The threat of it can be deployed to coerce women to behave in a certain way. A woman giving evidence to the Birthrights inquiry on racial injustice in maternity care was threatened with the removal of her baby if she continued to bedshare: '[They said] "If you do it again I will report you to social services and they will take the baby from you because you're not taking proper care of the baby, you're not keeping her in the cot."'[95]

The sanction of unmothering is also an internalised mechanism of control which ensures that women endeavour to conform to Good Mother norms. In her memoir on postnatal depression, the writer Emma Jane Unsworth observes:

> There are two great underlying fears for mothers, I think, and these ultimate fears inform every attempt to avoid shame and judgement: your baby is going to die, or (worse, somehow, socially) your baby is going to be taken away. It is from that fearful bedrock that we are frightened, harassed and bullied into conforming.[96]

When the writer Kirsty Logan had her mental health assessed as 'amber' rather than 'green' during an antenatal appointment, her thoughts immediately turned to unmothering: 'You think they'll take the baby. You smile at [the midwife], trying to be good good good, trying to be nice nice nice, and you go home and you lie in bed and stare at the ceiling and worry.'[97]

The fear of unmothering is a thread running through research among new mothers. An English qualitative study, which explored support for parents of excessively crying babies, found that women were reluctant to seek help about crying for fear of their babies being taken away.[98] A survey of 1,547 Netmums users who had experienced perinatal mental health problems found that most who discussed their wellbeing with a health professional were not completely honest (46%) or hid their illness altogether

(18%). A third (34%) of these women did so because they were worried about their baby being removed.[99] In qualitative research among new mothers in the UK with perinatal anxiety, women were hesitant to get professional help because they did not want to be considered a bad mother and some were afraid of their baby being taken away.[100] The same fears were found in research among ethnic minority women in the UK with perinatal mental health conditions and migrant women with depression in Canada, the US, the UK and Australia.[101] A migrant woman living in Canada disclosed:

> My biggest concern is that people will think I'm crazy or that I'm not normal and then they're going to come to the conclusion that I'm not able to take care of my child and then they're going to take my child from me. That's the biggest reason why I didn't go to seek any help.[102]

These fears of disclosing difficulties are shaped by deeply held cultural views about motherhood, which draw much of their strength from the myth of the natural. This myth works hand in hand with unmothering to enforce Good Mother norms.

It's Only Natural

Dr Spock told mothers to 'be natural and comfortable, and enjoy your baby'.[103] Kate Manne identifies narratives about women's natural preferences and abilities as a key mechanism used in support of women's subordination as givers.[104] Depicting motherhood as natural is a powerful instrument in circumscribing how mothers feel and behave. Women are naturally nurturing and maternal. Looking after children is rewarding and pleasurable. We want to be with our babies all the time and are happy to devote all our energies to our children. The myth of the natural is a strong pillar in Good Mother myths. Women with ambivalent or negative emotions are unnatural and must be ill or just plain bad.

Associating women with nature has deep cultural and histori-cal roots. In both Western and non-Western cultures, nature has traditionally been cast as feminine. We talk of Mother Nature and Mother Earth. In Latin and European languages, nature is a feminine noun.[105] 'Natural' also blurs into the animalistic. As Patricia Hill Collins has highlighted, portraying Black and Brown people as more 'natural' and animal-like, and therefore less human, has undergirded systems of domination such as slavery and colonialism.[106]

The ease with which 'nature' can be invoked to justify power structures was highlighted by the philosophers John Stuart Mill and Harriet Taylor. *The Subjection of Women* (1869), authored by Mill but heavily influenced by Taylor's thinking, asks: 'Was there ever any domination which did not appear natural to those who possessed it?'[107] What is customary is conflated with 'nature': 'So true is it that unnatural generally means only uncustomary, and that everything which is usual appears natural. The sub-jection of women to men being a universal custom, any departure from it quite naturally appears unnatural.'[108]

Portraying current social norms as 'natural' is a spurious defence of challenges to the status quo. The French scientist Gustave Le Bon wrote in 1879:

The day when, misunderstanding the inferior occupations which nature has given her, women leave the home and take part in our battles; on this day a social revolution will begin and everything that maintains the sacred ties of the family will disappear.[109]

Le Bon had no qualms about calling women 'inferior' but, over time, arguments have shifted away from women's 'natural' sub-ordination and the focus is now more on our 'natural' impulses and preferences. Silvia Federici observed in her 1975 book *Wages against Housework* how housework has been 'transformed into a natural attribute of our female physique and personality, an internal need, an aspiration, supposedly coming from the depth of our female character'.[110]

Similar claims are made about motherhood. The historian Jessica Martucci charts the development of the ideology of natural motherhood in post-war America. She identifies its central tenet to be that 'natural instincts of both an emotional and a physical nature govern maternal behavior and infant development'. She argues that the ideological framework of natural motherhood exerts a strong influence on 'mothers, policy makers, and health care providers whether they choose to embrace the ideology or not'.[111] As we shall see in later chapters, this ideology has shaped attitudes towards attachment theory, birth and breastfeeding, leaving women whose actions, choices and feelings do not fit certain norms at risk of being censured for being 'unnatural'.

'Natural' is still used to justify women being disadvantaged. The economist Linda Scott highlights how the gender pay gap is justified as the outcome of women's naturally made choices, rather than the result of discrimination and structural barriers. She quotes an article by the writer Tim Worstall in *Forbes* to make her point:

> It appears to be down to the different reactions of men and women to becoming a parent. Which, given that being a mammalian and viviparous species is pretty much central to the experience of being human means that the gender pay gap just might be one of those things not amenable to having a solution.[112]

What a convenient get out.

The concept of 'nature' derives much of its power from its strong moral undertones, particularly its association with purity and innocence. It is embraced as a bulwark against what is wrong with modern life. As the sociologist Charlotte Faircloth points out, 'natural' suggests something which is normal, right, non-artificial, traditional and instinctive.[113] People have been shown to favour items described as natural in many domains, including food, medicine, beauty products and even cigarettes.[114]

Put simply, 'nature' is hard to argue with. Courses of action that are described as natural are seen as more desirable than those regarded as unnatural. For instance, solutions to climate change that are framed as natural are more likely to be acceptable.[115] This was evident in a public deliberation about carbon capture storage which I worked on. Participants who were strongly opposed to this approach to reducing carbon emissions called it 'unnatural' to characterise it as dirty, expensive and dangerous.[116] The philosopher and historian Élisabeth Badinter describes nature as 'a decisive argument for imposing laws or dispensing advice'. She goes on to say: 'It is an ethical touchstone, hard to criticise and overwhelming all other considerations.'[117]

But there is an obvious flaw in automatically associating nature with something good. Tsunamis, tornadoes, snake venom and deadly nightshade are all natural. As the writer Eula Biss points out, 'the use of natural as a synonym for good is almost certainly a product of our profound alienation from the natural world'.[118]

The concept of nature draws on a sense of inevitability, as well as morality. It is positioned as something that just *is*, which cannot be questioned or rejected. The need to resist this myth was one of the central insights of the philosopher Simone de Beauvoir. She wrote 'a natural condition seems to defy change. In truth, nature is no more an immutable given than is historical reality.'[119] To return to Mill and Taylor's point, we should not confuse what is customary with 'nature'. As the historian Ludmilla Jordanova puts it, 'what appears natural is in fact a social-cum-cultural construct'.[120]

How mutable concepts like nature and instinct are is illustrated by the academic Celia Stendler's 1950 study of child-rearing advice in three popular American women's magazines from 1890 to 1940. She maps the shift from moralism (inculcating good character by example) to Watsonian behaviourism (moulding character through strict routines) and then Freudianism (fostering good emotional health). She concludes her review with a warning to be wary of 'mother's instinct' because this 'has had radically different meanings for practice during the past sixty years'.[121]

The concept of nature is not only powerful because it can be used to prescribe what mothers should do and feel. It can also be, as Charlotte Faircloth has observed in her research with mothers, a potential shield for women against scrutiny and judgement. Faircloth argues that justifying behaviour or choices on the grounds of nature or science (which we will look at in the next chapter) can provide women with 'a sort of relief from the constant requirement of accountability. Each of these strategies, albeit in different ways, forecloses further probing.'[122] The protagonist of *Soldier Sailor*, Claire Kilroy's wonderful novel on early motherhood, cites research studies when her husband criticises her mothering: 'I was on safe ground quoting infant studies . . . If there was one thing he couldn't refute, it was an infant study, having never read one.'[123]

Women can, and do, use science and the concept of 'nature' to defend themselves from Good Mother myths. The sociologist Patricia Hamilton highlights what she calls the currency of 'nature'. Black mothers in Britain and Canada participating in her research used this currency to resist oppressive narratives about Black mothering, as well as to justify parenting choices such as bedsharing. She draws our attention to the contrast between the stereotype of the naturally capable attachment mother from an imagined Africa and the way Black mothers are pathologised in the West. Both of these stereotypes are harmful. As Hamilton points out, while one demonises, the other dehumanises by portraying maternal practices as unthinking and driven by 'primitive' traditions.[124]

Even though motherhood is portrayed as natural and instinctive, women are not allowed to just get on with it. The contradiction that women are held to be naturally capable of mothering but in need of expert guidance has been highlighted by many.[125] It is another double bind. What mothers do is unthinking – it comes naturally – but our efforts are inadequate and cannot be trusted so we need to be told what to do. It's one of the ways in which women are set up to fail by Good Mother myths.

It also helps to explain the paradox that motherhood is both revered and undervalued – if we're just following our animal instincts, why should we get any credit? The sociologist Val Gillies makes the point that intense maternal labour is 'naturalised to the point of invisibility'.[126] What mothers do is taken for granted. This fits a neoliberal political agenda which seeks to whittle away public services. Patricia Hamilton highlights how 'women's "natural" proclivities for child-rearing can be cited as justification for the withdrawal of supportive structures and resources'. She notes that for Black women in particular, these arguments can be bolstered by the stereotype of the 'strong Black woman', which is used to justify withholding healthcare or support.

The myth of the natural tramples over women's agency and disregards our free will. If mother love is natural and instinctual, something that happens automatically, this discounts what the historian Marga Vicedo describes as 'the result of personal choice, intelligent decisions, or dutiful sacrifice'.[127] Claims that mothering is biologically driven, or making comparisons with animals, diminish women and their humanity. As Élisabeth Badinter put it, magnificently, we women are *not* chimpanzees.[128]

The archetype of the natural mother also fuels misogyny. Siri Hustvedt contrasts the 'perfect, caring, sacrificing, loving natural mother' (a being which has never existed) with 'the rejecting, selfish, unnatural mother who seeks power'. She goes on to observe that the 'scary, potentially abandoning mother must be punished. She is the source of male and female moral outrage.'

Hustvedt recalls being on the receiving end of some moral outrage herself when she forgot to strap her almost two-year-old daughter into a buggy as they went down an escalator. Hustvedt grabbed her daughter as she lurched forwards. This was witnessed by a businessman in front of her on the escalator:

He gave me a look I have never forgotten. It was a look of disgust, and the shame I felt was so bruising I have never shared this story with anyone until now. In his eyes I saw myself: a monster of negligence, the bad mother. It has taken me years to understand that the man on the escalator was an incarnation of the violent *moral* feelings in the culture directed at mothers. He made no move to block my child's potential fall. He showed no sympathy for my terror or subsequent relief. He was a figure of pure, brutal judgment.[129]

Moral outrage against 'unnatural' mothers permeates our culture. It can emanate from women as well as men, as Hustvedt notes. It helps explain why women can face harsh judgements and mistreatment from other women when they birth and feed their babies, issues which will be explored in later chapters.

Mothering Is Multifaceted – and Contingent

The myth of the natural presents motherhood as universal, detaching mothering from any context and providing moral imperatives to shame women into behaving in certain ways. But motherhood is shaped by the world we live in, both our individual circumstances and the social, economic and cultural forces that determine the texture of our lives.

The myth of the natural also ignores the wide range of feelings women have towards their children and the different ways in which mothers have cared for their babies over history. In her book *Mother: An Unconventional History*, the historian Sarah Knott argues powerfully for remembering the past:

> Historical forgetting leaves holes in the fabric that binds us. Things that seem natural only by force of repetition too easily take on a false status. Appeals to old, mistaken certainties, or to universals, stand uncorrected. How things are now too readily become how things were and should always be. It's not healthier to forget, to lose the past: historical remembering makes matters bigger and more open-ended.[130]

If we take a broader historical and cultural perspective, we can challenge Good Mother myths. We see that mothers are not inevitably the main carers of babies and children. There is not, and there has never been, a universal pattern of human care. African hunter-gatherers are sometimes portrayed as the single ancestral population from which we are all descended, but the anthropologists Sarah and Robert LeVine highlight wide variations in care shaped by different hunting and gathering patterns.[131]

It makes absolutely no evolutionary sense for there to be just one optimal pattern of care. As the paleoanthropologist Ian Tattersall points out, in evolution the important thing is not to be optimised for *anything*, simply to be good enough to get by in whatever circumstances present themselves.[132] Flexibility in child-rearing has enabled humans to survive and thrive in many different times and places. Anthropologist Sarah Hrdy observes that primates also have varied patterns of care and that the continuous care-and-contact mothering which is often associated with primates (and used to validate attachment theory as we shall see in a later chapter) is 'a last resort for primate mothers who lack safe and available alternatives'.[133]

Mothers spending all, or most, of their time with their young children without the support or company of others is a cultural and historical anomaly. A review of ethnographic studies conducted in 186 societies found that in only 3% were children almost exclusively cared for by their mother in the first year. This is similar to the proportion of societies (5%) where mothers provided half or less of the care. The most common pattern was the mother principally providing care with others in *minor* roles (44%), followed by the mother as the principal carer and others having *important* roles (34%). In early childhood (that is, from age one to the age of four or five), the role of the mother recedes. There are no recorded instances of children being almost exclusively cared for by their mother in any of the 186 societies. In only 19% did children spend their time principally with their mother. Young children were instead looked after by siblings, peers, older children and other adults.[134]

'Whoever can most easily be spared from more important tasks will take care of the child' is the rule of thumb in many societies the anthropologist David Lancy observes. Mothers are often too busy. The ethnographic record shows that in most societies women continue working throughout their pregnancy and start working again shortly after birth. Mothers are, in Lancy's words, often 'a critical contributor to the household economy'.[135] It is a Good Mother myth that working mothers are a modern phenomenon. For example, in *Double Lives: A History of Working Motherhood*, the historian Helen McCarthy recounts how Victorian and Edwardian mothers worked in factories, laundries, shops, fields and private homes.[136] In *Labor of Love, Labor of Sorrow*, the historian Jacqueline Jones describes how Black women in America have 'a long history of combining paid labour with domestic obligations'.[137]

What has been called a 'cooperative breeding' model helps explain why humans are able to combine relatively short birth intervals with a relatively long period of children being dependent.[138] The 'cooperative breeding' model relies on alloparents (from the Greek 'allo' meaning 'other than'). That is to say, anyone other than parents or siblings who helps rear a child.[139] Related to this, the 'grandmother hypothesis' provides an explanation for why women live long beyond their reproductive years, a trait not seen among primates. Daughters who were assisted by grandmothers, for instance through the provision of food or caring for infants, could have more children. Natural selection therefore favoured longer-living women.[140]

Where care isn't available, other strategies have to be employed. For example, in seventeenth-century Europe, young children from peasant and artisanal families were swaddled tightly and hung on hooks to prevent accidents while both parents were working.[141] Studies of American mothers conducted in the early twentieth century found that many took their children to work. Factory workers brought babies and preschool children to the factory. Agricultural workers put their babies in boxes, baskets or canvas tents in the fields and let older children play nearby. Some mothers left their children at home and checked in on them during the day.[142]

As well as there being nothing inevitable about how women care for their babies, it is also not guaranteed that they will do so at all. David Lancy notes that 'surveys of ethnographic and historical records affirm that the elimination of infants by abortion and infanticide is nearly a cultural universal'.[143] For instance, the exposure of unwanted babies in Greco-Roman antiquity was 'widespread' and was even legal in Imperial Rome until it was abolished by Emperor Valentinian in the third century.[144]

Eight centuries later, the abandonment of babies was institutionalised in Europe. The first foundling home is thought to have been established in 1198 by Pope Innocent III, who was said to be concerned by the number of infants being drowned in the Tiber River. Foundling wheels installed at churches or hospitals enabled parents to hand their babies over by placing them on a wheel which was turned to transport them into the building.

The historian David Kertzer recounts how the use of foundling homes became widespread in Florence and Milan in particular. By the 1830s, almost half of all children baptised in Florence were abandoned. In Milan in the mid-nineteenth century, almost all illegitimate children and a third of all legitimate children born in the city were left at the foundling home, Pia Casa. It seems one reason the practice was popular was because it was so straightforward. Babies could be left anonymously and parents were able to reclaim them without being punished or asked to repay expenses. Many parents did later try to retrieve their children – if they had not died, as many did – which could be as late as the age of five. When a London foundling home briefly adopted a similar system in the eighteenth century, Kertzer notes that 'vast numbers' of babies were left there.[145]

Wet nursing was also common in Europe for centuries. Wet nurses did more than breastfeed; babies were sent to live with them. For instance, Charles-Maurice de Talleyrand-Périgord, the wily diplomat whose career prospered through the reign of three kings, the French Revolution and Napoleon, was handed over to a wet nurse straight after his baptism on the day of his birth in 1754. His wet nurse looked after him in her home in a Paris suburb for more than four years. His mother did not visit him once and was unaware of Talleyrand's club foot. He may have been born with it or it may have been the result of an accident (he was said to have fallen off a chest of drawers).

We know how widespread the use of wet nurses was in France because it was meticulously documented by the state. By the eighteenth century, children of all classes were routinely placed in the care of wet nurses. In Paris in 1780, 19,000 of 21,000 children born that year were dispatched to the countryside. As late as 1907, nearly 80,000 of the newborns from large cities were sent away.[146]

Evidence from diaries and autobiographies suggests that wet nursing was also common in England, particularly in the London area, during the sixteenth and seventeenth centuries.[147] Jane Austen's mother's normal practice was to hand over her babies at around three months old to be looked after by a woman in her Hampshire village. Each child was returned home after a year or so, when it was regarded as old enough to be easily managed.[148]

Incidentally, the philosopher Jean-Jacques Rousseau's crusade against wet nursing is a glorious blend of mother blaming, spurious invocations of nature and rank hypocrisy. In *Emile* (1762), his influential treatise on education, he claimed that women refusing to breastfeed their children had resulted in national depravity. He urged: 'Let mothers deign to nurse their children. Morals will reform themselves, nature's sentiments will be awakened in every heart, the state will be repeopled.'[149] However, he abandoned his own five children in foundling homes.

In *The Myth of Motherhood*, Élisabeth Badinter explores why babies were left at foundling homes, given to wet nurses or led 'to the cemetery by the quickest route' in a series of steps 'winked at by society'. For the poorest families in French society, the considerations were economic: 'A new baby was a threat to the parents' very survival.' For women from well-to-do classes, different factors came into play: 'It seems they considered [raising children] an unworthy occupation and chose to get rid of the burden.' As Badinter concludes, 'mother love cannot be taken for granted'.[150]

The Heavy Weight of Good Mother Myths

Siri Hustvedt draws our attention to 'the "very happy mom" . . . an imaginary static being, a maternal figment used as a gilded hammer to beat the real mother into shape'.[151] A pervasive element of Good Mother myths is that good mothers are happy mothers and happy mothers are good mothers ('happy mother, happy baby' goes the adage).

Experts in the twentieth century presumed that child-rearing is pleasurable. For instance, in the 1935 advice manual *The Family Book*, which we met earlier in this chapter, mothers are described as 'happy slaves' who revel in their children.[152] Dr Spock counselled mothers to enjoy their baby – 'that's how he'll grow up best'.[153]

'A unit of mutual pleasure giving' was how the psychologist Penelope Leach described parents and children in her best-selling manual *Baby and Child: From Birth to Age Five* which was first published in 1977. She told women that their emotions and needs are inseparable from their child's:

> Your interests and hers are identical . . . If you make happiness for her, she will make happiness for you. If she is unhappy, you will find yourselves unhappy as well, however much you want or intend to keep your feelings separate from hers . . . Fun for her is fun for you.[154]

Mothers who were unhappy were assumed to be unwell. A disease model emerged during the second half of the twentieth century in popular magazines and advice books to explain any emotional difficulties mothers experienced. As the psychologists Lisa Held and Alexandra Rutherford drily observe, this 'did little to foster a cultural climate open to exploring a more nuanced, multi-layered motherhood narrative'. Throughout this period, the message was that mothers should not feel negative emotions, and, if they did, it was because something was wrong with the mother rather than motherhood itself.[155]

These beliefs still have strong currency. As we have seen, Siri Hustvedt highlights the moral outrage mothers can be subjected to. But the institution of motherhood – and the Good Mother myths that underpin it – is also, as Hustvedt says, 'a weapon that strikes mothers from the inside as shame or guilt'.[156] Women can feel like bad, abnormal or inadequate mothers if they have negative feelings about motherhood, find it difficult to cope, or feel they are falling short in some way.

These feelings of guilt, shame and inadequacy can make women miserable and ill. There is some evidence that women who have idealised and unforgiving standards of motherhood are at a greater risk of depression and anxiety. An American study of 383 pregnant women and new mothers found that those who agree with statements such as 'good mothers always put their baby's needs first' and 'if I make a mistake, people will think I am a bad mother' are more likely to experience depressive symptoms and perinatal anxiety.[157] A Portuguese study of 262 new mothers made the same link.[158] A survey of 631 users of Mumsnet (a UK parenting forum) who had experienced postnatal depression asked which factors had contributed to their depression. Pressure to be a perfect mother came top, selected by 65%, followed by a bad or traumatic birth experience (56%).[159]

The disparity between the myths and reality of motherhood can be overwhelming. 'Crushed maternal role expectations' was a key theme in the nursing academic Elizabeth Mollard's meta-synthesis of twelve qualitative studies on postnatal depression among women from several different countries, including the US and the UK. A 'good' mother was seen to be happy, self-less and patient; women felt like a 'bad' mother if they did not feel this way.[160] This echoes what the nursing academic Cheryl Beck found a decade earlier in her meta-synthesis of eighteen studies on postnatal depression among women in the US, the UK, Australia and Canada: 'Conflicting expectations and experiences of motherhood led them down the path to becoming overwhelmed, perceiving themselves as failures as mothers, and bearing a suffocating burden of guilt.'[161]

New mothers with perinatal anxiety who participated in a UK qualitative study said they felt under a great deal of pressure to be the 'perfect mum' and to do 'the right thing'. The researchers observed that this 'often equated to adhering to perceived societal norms, such as natural birth and breastfeeding'. There will be more on both in Chapters 3 and 4. The study noted that women felt 'an overwhelming sense of guilt and failure when they did not adhere to these societal scripts and fulfil the expectations they held about motherhood, often despite realising that these notions were unrealistic'.[162] A common theme in these studies is that women recognise that the standards they are holding themselves to are unrealistic and unattainable, but still blame themselves for being bad mothers.

Apprehension about being judged a bad mother can leave women feeling isolated and fearful about seeking support. 'Going into hiding' was a key theme Mollard identified in her meta-synthesis. Women felt compelled to present the façade of a good mother, while feeling like a fraud on the inside. So they withdrew from the outside world.[163] In a meta-synthesis of twenty-four qualitative studies exploring women's attitudes towards seeking help for perinatal psychological distress, the researchers found that women 'judged themselves harshly'. They regarded distress as a sign of weakness and felt under pressure to conform to ideal standards of motherhood.[164]

For women more vulnerable to scrutiny and judgement, the fear of being judged a bad mother can be particularly acute. We see this in studies of disabled mothers. In her 1997 study among disabled mothers in England, the sociologist Carol Thomas found that the women were afraid of being seen as inadequate mothers and went to great lengths to present themselves as managing to cope. This was 'often at significant personal cost in terms of comfort and emotional and physical well-being'. An example was making sure their home was always clean. One woman recalled:

> I would love to have those months again cos I was so scared, tidying the house cos I knew somebody was coming who was from authority . . . I was too busy doing jobs rather than enjoying him and relaxing.[165]

The researcher Julia Daniels reflects that disabled mothers 'are barred from the sacred hallow of motherhood'. She feared asking for help because of being judged as an incapable mother and inviting scrutiny from child protection services:

> So I pretended, I passed, I masked. This turned a potentially positive experience into the start of a downward emotional spiral. In a sense, the only real risk came from the lack of adequate support in my environment, and the anxiety of surveillance – both attributable to living in a 'disablist world'.[166]

As this illustrates, women who do not fit Good Mother archetypes can find the weight of Good Mother myths especially hard to bear. The writer Aly Windsor recounts the 'endless pressure' she felt when her son was a baby, of 'the constant feeling that I should be in control of all aspects of my child's development, that he was crying or not sleeping or not eating the right foods because I was failing at my job'. She did not want to share her difficulties with others in case of being labelled a bad mother: 'I especially couldn't bear to risk revealing weakness to people who thought that, as one half of a same-sex couple, I should never have had a child in the first place.'[167]

Patricia Hamilton observes that Black women face 'additional, racially specific pressure' on top of the intense scrutiny of child-rearing choices that all women can encounter. One of the women in her study remarked:

> When it comes to parenting and I think most Black people have always heard the same, you know, you have to be twice as good . . . to get half of what they have . . . it affects my parenting, whether I want it to or not.[168]

Good Mother myths are extremely potent. They draw their strength from women's love for their children. It is very difficult to question, ignore or defy prescriptions about mothering if we are told this will harm our children. Guilt is a key mechanism at work here. As Adrienne Rich observes, 'guilt is one of the most powerful forms of social control of women; none of us can be entirely immune to it'.[169] Guilt is used to contain and corral mothers. It has been weaponised to keep women focused on their apparent maternal failings, rather than the ways in which they and their children are being failed by society.

Good Mother myths are bad for women's emotional health and deny them permission to look after their own needs or process the emotions they feel. It is a double bind that Good Mother myths simultaneously make women unhappy while requiring that mothers must be happy. Intensive mothering – and its mantra of the 'more the better' – sets impossibly high standards for women and devalues the care and love mothers give. It is the latest iteration of mother blame and undergirds inequality and racism. It is only because the role of women as givers is so deeply culturally embedded that the logical absurdity of the 'more the better' is not even questioned.

The myth of the natural is an important pillar in Good Mother myths, obliging mothers to give everything of themselves and to do so happily. Women's status as givers means that what mothers do is not valued because it is taken for granted. Mothers who do not conform to Good Mother norms, especially those more liable to be judged harshly because of race, sexuality, class or disability, are deemed to be unnatural. The spectre of unmothering casts a dark shadow.

The myth of the natural works hand in hand with another important pillar of Good Mother myths – science. We shall turn to this next. As Patricia Hamilton observes, 'scientific motherhood is draped in the language of "nature."' Both seek to tell women what to do, drawing on deep reservoirs of maternal love and care. Both claim to be authoritative. Both are deployed unfairly and unjustly. Motherdom means challenging both the myth of the natural and bad science.

2

Why Science Can't Talk

'Put the cellphone away!' urges a press release from the University of California, Irvine. 'Fragmented baby care can affect brain development.'[1] This directive was issued on the basis of a study conducted with six male rats (female rats were originally part of the experiment but were later excluded, with no reason given).

Warning women off cellphones is a classic example of using research to tell mothers what to do. It is also a stark illustration of how directives can be issued on the flimsiest of evidence. Animal studies may suggest potential lines of enquiry for research, but they don't tell us anything definitive about humans. We women are not chimpanzees, to repeat Élisabeth Badinter's point. And our children are not rats either. These may be obvious points, but, as we shall see, using animal studies is a favourite trick of people who deploy science to moralise about motherhood.

In this particular study, half of the pups were placed with mothers in cages with limited bedding and nesting materials, the other half in cages with sufficient bedding. The male rats (not the females remember) were then observed a couple of months after birth, which is adolescence in rat terms. In five out of six measures of peer play, the two groups were similar. However, the male rats raised in the impoverished cages spent less time playing with peers (31% of their time versus 45%). They also drank less sucrose than the other group, although for both groups the majority of their total liquid intake was sucrose. The press release misleadingly claims that this group 'exhibited little interest in sweet foods or peer play, two independent measures of the ability to experience pleasure'.

The research paper attributed the differences in sucrose intake and time playing with peers to maternal care. This was despite the fact that on several measures the quantity and quality of maternal care were the same, a finding the researchers revealingly describe as 'unexpected'. However, maternal care was deemed to be fragmented and unpredictable because individual bouts of grooming were shorter and the sequence of nurturing behaviours was less likely to follow the same order. The paper concluded, 'We *speculate* [my italics] that patterns of maternal-derived sensory input, specifically unpredictable and fragmented patterns, might influence the maturation of emotional systems within the developing brain.'[2]

Dr Tallie Baram, a developmental neuroscientist who was one of the study's authors, was unequivocal in the press release though. She claimed that the study 'shows that it is not *how much* maternal care that influences adolescent behaviour but the avoidance of fragmented and unpredictable care that is crucial'. She then added, 'We might wish to turn off the mobile phone when caring for baby and be predictable and consistent.'

University press releases routinely overplay research findings. One study examining 462 press releases from 20 leading UK research universities found that 40% of the press releases contained more direct advice than the journal article, 33% were more likely to draw causal statements from correlational results (more on this shortly) and 36% contained exaggerated inferences to humans from animal research.[3] These press releases usually determine how studies are covered in the media. A Dutch study examining 129 university press releases found that where these carried exaggerated conclusions, 92% of news articles covering the study included the same exaggeration. If there was no exaggeration in the press release, only 6% of news articles contained exaggerations.[4]

There are obvious incentives in overstating research findings to make them more newsworthy. In our study of male rats, the press release did its job and Dr Baram's warnings about the dangers of using mobile phones were dutifully reported. *Time* ran a piece entitled 'Cell-Phone Distracted Parenting Can Have Long-Term Consequences'.[5] While journalists are sometimes criticised for not being scientifically literate, we can hardly blame them if universities keep peddling flimsy findings.

Why Fish Need to Notice Water

The way in which the rat research was conducted, interpreted and reported illustrates how science is used to dispense directives to mothers. The assumption, never questioned, is that everything measured is related to mothering. Even if we believe that it is legitimate to issue edicts about human behaviour on the basis of research with a few male rats, the study is arguably as much about growing up in an impoverished environment. But this explanation doesn't fit the narrative of mother blame.

The study's findings are interpreted in a way that breaks one of the fundamental tenets of science; correlation is not causation. In other words, associations in the data between one thing (for instance how a mother behaves) and another (a child's development) do not prove that one caused the other. But, as we shall see, assumptions about cause and effect abound in research about mothers and their children.

Why is this so pervasive? It is partly because of our need to find explanations for what happens. The psychologist Daniel Kahneman highlights our predilection for causal thinking and our inability to identify complexity and randomness: 'We are pattern seekers, believers in a coherent world'.[6] Tyler Vigen pokes fun at this tendency in his book *Spurious Correlations* – for instance, rises in the per capita consumption of cheese in the US correlate with increases in the number of people who died by becoming tangled in their bedsheets.[7]

Correlations are easy to find in a study with lots of measures. Charles Babbage, best known for inventing the concept of a computer memorably described this process as cooking the data in 1830: 'If a hundred observations are made, the cook must be very unhappy if he cannot pick out fifteen or twenty which will do for serving up.'[8]

Cutting the data in different ways expands the likelihood of finding correlations. For instance, looking separately at girls and boys immediately doubles the possibilities. The psychology researcher Judith Harris calls this tactic 'divide and conquer'.[9] We see all of this at play in the rat study, where the female rats are discarded from the analysis and maternal care is measured in seven ways, with a story spun on the basis of differences in only two of these measures.

Social scientists Joseph Simmons, Leif Nelson and Uri Simonsohn managed to 'prove' that listening to the Beatles song 'When I'm Sixty-Four' could make someone younger.[10] They did so to illustrate how it is possible to play around with the data until you get a statistically significant finding (that is, the results are not explainable by chance alone). This practice is known variously as data dredging, significance chasing, significance questing, selective inference and 'p-hacking' (p-tests are used to determine the significance of the results).[11] The more significance tests that are carried out, the higher the chance of false positives. This was demonstrated in one famous experiment when scientists scanned the brain of a dead salmon while showing it photographs – they found a statistically significant response in 16 out of 8,064 points in the brain.[12]

The statistician and writer Nate Silver highlights the importance of distinguishing *noise* (random patterns in the data) from *signals* (an indication of an underlying truth or meaningful information).[13] For instance, large observational studies found an association between vitamin E and a lower likelihood of heart disease. When this was investigated in randomised control trials, giving people vitamin E made no difference to their chances of dying from heart disease.[14]

Even if an association is meaningful rather than random statistical noise, we need to think carefully about which way the relationship works, as well as what the other factors shaping it are. So mother–child relationships must be seen in a wider context to understand the impact of factors such as poverty, racism and social class. Parents and children share genes, making it tricky to untangle genetic influences and how children are brought up. The relationship between parents and children works in both directions. For instance, a Canadian study of 628 parents found an association between children's behavioural problems at the age of three and binge drinking and coercive parenting (shouting, getting angry, hitting the child) two years later when the children were aged five. The researchers suggested that the stresses of dealing with their children's behaviour could have contributed to parents' drinking and harsh parenting.[15] Rigorous research recognises and tries to account for these complexities. But a failure to recognise children's agency and influence is a common blind spot in research about parents.

And there are blind spots galore in research involving mothers and children. Dorothy Bishop is a developmental neuropsychologist, but also a passionate and eloquent advocate of challenging bad science. She highlights the role of confirmation bias in science, the inclination 'to seek out and remember evidence that supports a preferred viewpoint'. This contributes to what she calls the 'entrenchment of false theories' through biased literature reviews 'that put a disproportionate focus on findings that are consistent with the author's position'.

Bishop also calls out the tendency of researchers to 'converge on accepting the most obvious causal explanation, without considering lines of evidence that might point to alternative possibilities'. She gives the example of how many books there are at home predicting reading outcomes in children. This finding is typically explained as demonstrating that access to books at home positively influences children's reading. However, an alternative explanation is that parents and children share genetic risks for reading problems. The evidence for this is that children who are poor readers tend to have parents who are poor readers.[16]

The most obvious causal explanations are accepted because science is grounded in deeply held and often unexamined assumptions. The philosopher of science Thomas Kuhn described how scientists work to what he called 'community paradigms' which have an 'underlying body of rules and assumptions'.[17]

'The last thing a fish would ever notice would be water,' wrote the anthropologist Ralph Linton in 1936, which is another way of putting it.[18] Our underlying assumptions are either not recognised or regarded as just common sense. These assumptions shape every aspect of scientific enquiry, all the way from what is researched to how findings are analysed and disseminated.

Science derives its authority from its apparent objectivity. But science does not operate in a vacuum, and it is not objective. As the feminist philosopher Sandra Harding has argued, 'gender politics . . . can and often do shape every stage of scientific research'.[19] Philosopher of science Helen Longino explains that what she calls 'background assumptions' shape how evidence is gathered and interpreted. She argues that these assumptions may be unrecognised and therefore immune from scrutiny: 'If . . . we deny their existence, they become enshrined and all the more powerful for being invisible.'[20]

A good example of this is the assumption that males and females in forager societies have separate and gendered roles, leading to the well-known paradigm of men as hunters and women as gatherers. Cara Wall-Scheffler, a biological anthropologist, was struck by recent archaeological discoveries, such as a 9,000-year-old burial in the Andes, of women being buried with hunting tools.[21] Wall-Scheffler and a group of researchers re-analysed ethnographic data on sixty-three different foraging societies across the world and found that 79% had documentation on women hunting. In the forty-one societies where there was enough detail to ascertain this, this hunting was intentional in most cases (87%) rather than opportunistic. As the researchers conclude, it is about time that we reassessed 'man the hunter' narratives.[22]

Science Starts Talking: Scientific Sexism

Background assumptions are easier to recognise when we look to the past. In Victorian times, would-be scientific arguments were used to rationalise rigid gender roles. Women's development was said to be arrested in comparison to men's. Similar arguments were made about 'primitive' peoples and 'superior' Europeans; this was also the era of 'scientific racism'. Scientists such as Francis Galton (who coined the term 'eugenics') used measurements of the human body to rank different racial groups. The academic Anne McClintock describes how White women were 'seen as an inherently degenerate "race," akin in physiognomy to Black people and apes'. However, White middle-class women were regarded as higher up the evolutionary hierarchy than Black, Irish or Jewish men – and, of course, Black women were placed right at the bottom of the hierarchy.[23]

One reason given for women's arrested development was the need to preserve their energies for reproduction. This apparent logic was used to oppose female education, with doctors in the UK and the US arguing that women's brains and reproductive systems could not develop at the same time.[24] The philosopher and biologist Hebert Spencer cautioned that higher education would leave women unable to breastfeed and probably also infertile.[25] Eminent physician Henry Maudsley warned in his 1874 book *Sex in Mind and Education* that a hard-working schoolgirl may leave college 'a good scholar but a delicate and ailing woman . . . the special functions which have relation to her future offices as a woman . . . have been deranged at a critical time'. Maudsley marshalled both science and nature to argue against female education: 'In the long-run Nature, which cannot be ignored or defied with impunity, asserts its power; excessive losses occur.'[26]

Developments in scientific knowledge were interpreted through the lens of contemporary prejudices, sometimes comically so. George Romanes, an evolutionist, physiologist and early comparative psychologist, declared in 1887 that 'we must look the fact in the face . . . it must take many centuries for heredity to produce the missing five ounces of the female brain'. When scientists realised that women's brains are actually heavier than men's in relation to body weight, the argument changed. Women's proportionately larger brains demonstrated their childlike physiology.[27] As the historians Carroll Smith-Rosenberg and Charles Rosenberg put it in a 1973 paper, 'medical and scientific arguments formed an ideological system rigid in its support of tradition, yet infinitely flexible in the particular mechanisms which could be made to explain and legitimate woman's role'.[28]

There is, as the historian Cynthia Russett points out, a long history of scientific interest in women. But what was new about what Russett calls 'sexual science' was its attempts to be empirical and its assumption of authority. Science was given a voice which was used to tell women what to do: 'It spoke with the imperious tone of a discipline newly claiming, and in large measure being granted, decisive authority in matters social as well as strictly scientific.' But the apparent empiricism of 'sexual science' was deeply flawed. As the historian Jane Lewis notes, circular arguments were deployed – women were prevented from acquiring certain capacities and then science provided the justification for this on the basis that these capacities were 'naturally' absent. Influential thinkers such as Romanes, Spencer and other scientific authorities constructed, in the words of Russett, 'a feminine psyche very much in accord with prevailing cultural views of womanhood – gentle, emotional, nurturant, weak-willed, and dependent'.[29]

Women who behaved in ways at odds with cultural norms, such as smoking or using slang, were seen to be suffering from 'simple hysterical mania'.[30] Behaviour as diverse as reading, studying in excess, having a luxurious lifestyle, wearing improper clothing, or working long hours in a factory were deemed to produce 'weak and degenerate offspring'.[31] There are parallels with today, as we shall see, in the way that women are held responsible for damaging their babies' brains.

The Rise and Fall of the Bonding Myth

Scientists are widely trusted. My former employer Ipsos has been measuring how much the British public trusts different professions since 1983. According to the latest figures, 74% trust scientists to tell the truth, up eleven percentage points since 1997.[32] An Ipsos survey in twenty-one countries asked about the trustworthiness of eighteen professions. Scientists came second in the global average, just behind doctors, with 57% regarding them as trustworthy (politicians are at the bottom with 14%). In the US, scientists are third, just behind teachers and doctors.[33]

But there is more to it than this. Science can be presented as authoritative and unimpeachable. The psychologist Diane Eyer argues that we have made scientists into a modern clergy, interpreters of texts deriving from infallible authority.[34] Charlotte Faircloth makes a similar point: 'The use of "evidence" has reached the level of the quasi-religious; not in the sense that the beliefs are other-worldly (quite the opposite) but that they are held to be beyond the possibility of doubt and revered as truth.'[35]

Eyer's 1992 book *Mother-Infant Bonding: A Scientific Fiction* illustrates how flimsy scientific evidence that aligns with cultural ideals can be eagerly accepted. The story of the bonding myth is worth retelling. As the psychologist Ben Bradley observes, it is 'a myth that fully accords with tendencies for men to argue that women are better fitted than themselves to rear small babies, and to see a lack of mother-love as the main cause of children's problems'.[36] Eyer argues that one of the reasons for the potency of the bonding myth is because it supported deep-seated views on gender which were being challenged by the legal and economic gains women were making in the 1970s.

The bonding myth rests on a study of twenty-eight mothers and their newborn babies which was conducted by two paediatricians, Dr Marshall H. Klaus and Dr John H. Kennell. Half of the mothers and babies in the study had skin-to-skin contact at birth and additional contact over the next three days; the other half were separated after birth, as was the practice in American hospitals at the time. The babies were followed up after one month and then again at one, two and five years old. Mothering and infant development was deemed to be better in the extra contact group, even though the only difference at the age of two was that extended-contact mothers asked more questions and used fewer commands and at the age of five the extended-contact babies scored better on language tests.

Klaus and Kennell concluded in their influential 1976 book *Maternal-Infant Bonding: The Impact of Early Separation or Loss on Family Development* that 'there is a sensitive period in the first minutes and hours of life during which it is necessary that the mother and father have close contact with their neonate for later development to be optimal.'[37] Note the use of the word optimal here. As we saw in Chapter 1, this is now commonly bandied about as part of the ideology of intensive motherhood, and we shall consider it again. As I argue in the final chapter of this book, we need to fiercely reject the concept of 'optimal' as far as child-rearing is concerned.

The belief that there is a biologically based sensitive period after birth which shapes a baby's development was enthusiastically embraced in the US and beyond. An example is *Pregnancy and Parenthood,* a book published by the National Childbirth Trust in 1980 (the copy I have I inherited from my mum who used it in her work as a health visitor). It includes a whole section called 'Bonding' which said, 'recent research has demonstrated that this long-held feeling about the value of early holding of the newborn baby by his mother is founded on a good basis of fact.'[38]

However, Klaus and Kennell were making big claims on the basis of a tiny study of twenty-eight babies and subsequent research failed to replicate their results. Two different groups of researchers subjected bonding theory to detailed critiques, including cataloguing the methodological flaws in the original study of twenty-eight babies. Both groups of researchers concluded that there is no evidence to support bonding theory.[39]

Faced with this criticism, Klaus and Kennell rowed back. Reflecting on the claim that close contact after birth is required for optimal development, Dr Klaus is quoted in a 1983 interview as saying, 'I wish we'd never written the statement'.[40] In a piece published a year later, Klaus and Kennell reflected that part of the problem was the over-enthusiastic application of bonding theory: 'Unfortunately, some misinterpretations of studies of parent-to-infant attachment may have resulted from a too literal acceptance of the word *bonding*, suggesting that the speed of this reaction resembles that of epoxy glue.'[41]

But this is disingenuous. Klaus's and Kennell's study should have been treated with caution – an interesting hypothesis to further investigate – rather than swallowed whole as scientific truth. There is the muddling of correlation and causation – is it really plausible that any apparent differences between the two groups of children at the age of five could be explained by what happened a few moments after birth? And then there is the small number of babies involved in the research, a key reason why its results should have been treated with much more caution.

Beware Small Numbers and Weird Samples

The number of people taking part in a research study matters. With bigger sample sizes, results are less likely to be random chance. This can be illustrated by throwing a dice. If you roll a dice six times (as I just have), you are unlikely to roll a perfect 1, 2, 3, 4, 5 and 6. My numbers are 6, 5, 2, 6, 5, 5. This does not give me a very accurate picture of the dice – there are no 1s, 3s or 4s and half the rolls are 5s. When I roll the dice thirty-six times, the results are a better reflection of the dice, with most numbers rolled six or seven times. However, I rolled 6 eight times and 4 four times. If I ask an online generator to throw a dice 1,000 times, every number appears 16% or 17% of the time. I now have an accurate picture of the dice.

One of the things which surprised me when I started reading research papers about mothers and babies is how tiny the sample sizes often are (in Chapter 5, we will meet a legendary study involving only twenty-three babies). I have worked in market and social research for most of my professional life and sample sizes of 1,000 or 2,000 are the norm for a survey among a representative sample of the general public.

There are obvious reasons why it is challenging to conduct studies with that many mothers and children. But there is more to it than that. Daniel Kahneman and Amos Tversky coined the expression 'the Law of Small Numbers' to describe our tendency to assume that small samples (or fewer rolls of the dice) are as robust as larger samples (or more rolls of the dice).[42] Kahneman highlights our 'exaggerated faith' in small samples and attributes this to our tendency to jump to conclusions and our inability to grasp randomness.[43]

I was also taken aback by the sample design of many mother and baby studies. Sample design determines who takes part in a study and is fundamental to what conclusions (if any) can be drawn from it. 'A survey is only as good as its sample' was drilled into me at the start of my research career at MORI. George Gallup was the pioneer of opinion polling whose research famously predicted Franklin D. Roosevelt's victory in the 1936 American presidential election. He compared sampling to soup. If you have cooked a large pan of soup, you do not need to eat it all to see if it needs more salt – you just taste a spoonful. However, you must have given it a good stir so all the ingredients have an equal chance of being chosen.[44]

I'd take the analogy further – you need to be sure you've got the right ingredients in the soup before you start drawing conclusions from tasting it. A good example of a well-made soup is the

Millennium Cohort Study, which is following the lives of around 19,000 young people born in the UK at the turn of the century. It uses robust sampling strategies to ensure it is representative of the population and it has a large enough sample to allow comparisons between different groups, such as ethnic minority children.[45]

Most psychology studies use samples which, to use an acronym from a famous paper, are WEIRD; that is to say 'Western, Educated, Industrialised, Rich, and Democratic'. In this paper, the academics Joseph Henrich, Steven J. Heine and Ara Norenzayan analysed a comparative database from across the behavioural sciences and found that WEIRD populations are frequent outliers across a range of domains, such as visual perception, spatial reasoning, cooperation, moral reasoning and the heritability of IQ. They conclude: 'The findings suggest that members of WEIRD societies, including young children, are among the least representative populations one could find for generalising about humans.' Even within Western societies, study participants may not be representative, as they tend to be from higher income groups. Despite sampling 'from a thin slice of humanity' as the paper puts it, researchers often draw more general conclusions about human behaviour.[46]

Small and WEIRD samples help explain why psychological studies are dogged by a lack of replicability. The Reproducibility Project, an undertaking involving over 270 researchers, conducted replications of 100 experimental and correlational studies published in three psychology journals. Almost all of the original studies (97 in total) had statistically significant results, but when they were repeated, only 39% did so. As the authors of the paper dryly noted 'humans desire certainty and science infrequently provides it.' They concluded that 'scientific progress is a cumulative process of uncertainty reduction that can only succeed if science itself remains the greatest sceptic of its explanatory claims.'[47]

The Power of Mother Love to Grow Brains?

Unfortunately, scepticism is often in short supply, and explanatory claims are swallowed whole. A good example of this is a study that was publicised with a press release entitled 'Mom's love good for child's brain'.[48] This American study of ninety-two children measured levels of maternal support between the ages of four to seven and then scanned the children's brains between the ages of seven to thirteen.[49] Maternal support was determined in a laboratory using 'the waiting task'. Children were required to wait for eight minutes before opening a brightly wrapped present within arm's reach. Researchers classified the strategies the parent used to help the child wait as supportive or non-supportive. The *Manual for the Waiting Task* used in the study is unpublished, so it is not possible to see on what basis parental behaviours are assessed and how the approach has been validated (if at all). But can we really get a handle on the extent of parental support in the early years from observing a few minutes of interaction in a laboratory? The lead researcher, Dr Joan Luby, is in no doubt about the validity of the test though, describing it as 'very objective' in the press release.

The researchers divided the children into four groups on the basis of high or low maternal support and depression severity. This appears to be because the relationship which the researchers found between maternal support and hippocampus volume only holds for children in the high maternal support/low depressive severity group. It's a good example of cooking the data. Frustratingly, the paper doesn't say how many children were in each group, although with an overall sample of ninety-two, the numbers will be low. There are no figures given – the results for the four groups are shown in a graph – but the differences appear to be in the region of 120–220 mm³ depending on the group. Should we be worried about these differences in hippocampus size? A much larger study of 1,099 children found 'marked variability in brain structure'.[50]

The researchers did acknowledge some limitations; maternal support was only measured earlier in childhood and not later on and the differences might be genetic. However, there is no discussion on whether obvious issues, such as weight, height and puberty (an important period of brain development as we shall see) could account for the differences in brain size. The children were aged between seven and thirteen years so there may have been considerable variation in these factors. There is also no discussion of whether the differences are just statistical noise (the paper doesn't mention whether other brain regions were scanned) or if they are actually meaningful.

Despite all these limitations, the researchers drew some unequivocal conclusions: 'The finding that early parenting support, a modifiable psychosocial factor, is directly related to healthy development of a key brain region known to impact cognitive functioning and emotion regulation opens an exciting opportunity to impact the development of children in a powerful and positive fashion.'

And, in a familiar pattern, the press release makes even more sweeping claims, with Dr Luby declaring: 'Having a hippocampus that's almost 10 percent larger just provides concrete evidence of nurturing's powerful effect.' Every time I read this sentence, I want to scream 'correlation is not causation'. But if Luby had been more circumspect, she would not be in a position to dish out this directive in the press release: 'Parents should be taught how to nurture and support their children. Those are very important elements in healthy development.'

The paper concludes by saying, 'This finding, *when* [my emphasis] replicated, would strongly suggest enhancement of public policies and programs that provide support and parenting education to caregivers early in development.' The assumption that the finding will be replicated is very telling. We are about as far from genuine scientific enquiry as it is possible to imagine. This is a matter of faith, not science.

Luby and her group of researchers did manage to replicate the findings – but only with some serious statistical jiggery pokery.

The subsequent study was among 127 children and looked at the relationship between increases in hippocampal volumes, which were measured three times across school age, and levels of maternal support at preschool and school age. The 'waiting task' was again used to ascertain maternal support at preschool age and the 'puzzle task' at school age. This involves the child completing a puzzle in a box, guided by their parent, without being able to see the pieces.

The researchers did not find any relationship between levels of support at school age and hippocampus size. So they cast their net wider and managed to find a link between preschool support and brain size by comparing children with maternal support one standard deviation *below* the mean and children with maternal support one standard deviation *above* the mean (a standard deviation is a measure of how spread out numbers are). No rationale is given for analysing the data in this way (it's not an approach to analysis I've ever come across). The research has the same flaws as the other study. Are the differences meaningful (the hippocampus increased by 1.31% in the first group and 2.70% in the second group), what about other factors such as weight and how much can two laboratory tasks actually tell us about how much nurturing children receive? All of these issues were again ignored and the researchers declared:

> These study findings provide, to our knowledge, the first evidence for the long-term effects of early maternal support on the development of the hippocampus through school age and early adolescence. They also suggest that maternal support during the preschool period may represent a sensitive period when these experiences have a uniquely powerful effect on brain development.[51]

The press release for the study, entitled 'Nurturing during preschool years boosts child's brain growth', went even further. It claimed that 'children whose mothers were nurturing during the preschool years . . . have more robust growth in brain structures associated with learning, memory and stress response than children with less supportive moms.'[52] The press release did its job, and the study was picked up by the media on both sides of the Atlantic.

'Why a mother's love really does matter: Nurturing helps children's brains grow at TWICE the rate of those who are "neglected"' was the headline of a *Daily Mail* piece. The article went on to claim: 'A mother's love could make a child's brain grow. Research found a key brain structure to grow more than twice as quickly in youngsters whose mothers were affectionate and supportive than those with cold and distant parents.'[53]

The Seductive Allure of Neuroscience

Why are we so willing to swallow such nonsense about children's brains? There is something about neuroscience which makes us particularly likely to trust it, a phenomenon which has been described as the 'seductive allure effect'.[54] A series of studies has demonstrated that we are more likely to believe faulty scientific explanations (for example, circular restatements) if they are accompanied by neuroscientific information.[55] One study found that bad explanations using neuroscience had more credibility than those deriving from natural sciences, such as chemistry, biology and the social sciences. The researchers speculate that part of the allure of neuroscience over and above other branches of science is that 'it allows the neat, tidy attribution to one causal source: the brain'.[56] This is the pattern seeking which, as we have seen, Daniel Kahneman warns us we are so susceptible to.

Neuroscience narratives have been enthusiastically adopted by political actors. The wagon started rolling in the 1990s. In his book *The Myth of the First Three Years*, the philosopher John Bruer relates how the report *Starting Points: Meeting the Needs of Our Youngest Children* sparked everything off. Published in 1994 by the Carnegie Corporation, it included a short section on brain development. In these paragraphs, the report argued that recent scientific findings demonstrated that the influence of the early environment on brain development is long-lasting. The report generated extensive media coverage as a result.[57]

Bruer's book explores the lack of scientific support for the idea that the first three years is uniquely important for brain development. One of the core arguments he takes on is that this is a period of peak synaptic density (that is, number of synapses per volume of brain tissue). But a high density of synapses in the brain continues well beyond age three (lasting until near puberty or beyond for some brain areas), and the formation of synapses appears to be under genetic control, rather than stimulation playing a fundamental role. Brain plasticity allows us to continue to acquire new knowledge and skills throughout our lives. London black cab drivers are a famous example of this. The test they have to pass to qualify, known as 'The Knowledge', requires memorising the name and location of every street and the shortest or quickest route to it within a six-mile radius of Charing Cross. In comparison to non-taxi drivers, black cab drivers have been found to have a larger hippocampus, a region of the brain associated with spatial navigation. Hippocampus volume was related to how long someone had been a cab driver, suggesting that the differences are due to the experience of driving.[58]

But the lack of strong evidence for the brain claims in *Starting Points* was neither here nor there. The report had hit upon fertile territory by providing scientific justification for deeply rooted beliefs which the psychologist Jerome Kagan has called 'infant determinism' – the view that 'experiences during the early years (especially the biological mother's affectionate care and interactive play with her infant) are the most potent force in shaping a life'.[59]

This ground has subsequently been tilled with great effectiveness by the Harvard Center on the Developing Child (established in 2006) and its related body, the National Scientific Council on the Developing Child (established in 2003). Both were founded by Jack Shonkoff, an academic paediatrician, not a neuroscientist.

These two institutions have been adept at popularising neuroscience through the use of what they call 'simplifying models' such as 'toxic stress' and 'serve and return'. These models are designed to 'reduce the complexity of a social or scientific concept to the form of a simple, concrete analogy or metaphor'. These models have been developed in partnership with communications specialists the FrameWorks Institute. They are honed through consultation and extensive research which tests them for their communicability. For instance, an initial simplifying model of 'chemicals in the brain' was reworked into 'toxic stress' because it was not powerful enough. The final stage of the testing is a quantitative phase, where brief exposures to various models are analysed in terms of their impact on selected policy preferences in order 'to determine whether they can bring people close to using scientific reasoning to think about proposed solutions'.

This is all set out in a paper written by Shonkoff and Susan Nall Bales, CEO of the FrameWorks Institute. The title of the paper is telling – *Science Does Not Speak for Itself: Translating Child Development Research for the Public and Its Policymakers*.[60] Shonkoff and Bales regard their approach as a means to giving a voice to science in the public domain.

In the paper, Shonkoff and Bales are at pains to stress the scientific credibility of what they call their core story of development, saying it is based on 'well-established, science-based principles'. However, they are guilty of some sleights of hand which are anything but science-based. They routinely apply animal research to humans on the (questionable) grounds that 'the development of animal brains follows comparable biological processes'. A common feature of neuroscience papers and books is making sweeping claims which are justified by footnotes citing animal studies. We have already seen some examples of this and there are more to come.

Brain claims jettison a core scientific principle by deliberately confusing probabilities with certainties. Shonkoff and Bales are open about this, attributing the power of their core story to 'the degree to which we describe causal mechanisms (not simply report statistical associations) in concrete terms that explain how early experience shapes brain architecture and developmental outcomes (both for good and for bad)'. For example, an influential 2007 paper *The Science of Early Childhood Development*, published by the National Scientific Council on the Developing Child claims (using the voice of science): 'Decades of research tell us that mutually rewarding interactions are essential prerequisites for the development of healthy brain circuits and increasingly complex skills.'[61]

But there are no certainties in science, as in life. The neuroscientist and philosopher Raymond Tallis labels descriptions of later behaviour as being 'hard-wired' by earlier experiences as pseudo-science. There is a higher probability that neglect leads to poor outcomes, but neglect does not automatically lead to delinquency or anything else.[62]

A basic rule of thumb of forecasting is that the longer the timescales, the trickier it is to predict the future. A huge amount can happen between the ages of three and adulthood. Later experiences can be good, bad or catastrophically awful. As other experiences pile up, the baby years fade away. As Jerome Kagan puts it in his critique of infant determinism:

> Both science and autobiography affirm that a capacity for change is as essential to human development as it is to the evolution of new species. The events of the opening years do start an infant down a particular path, but it is a path with an extraordinarily large number of intersections.[63]

Another sleight of hand is the failure to acknowledge that the brain claims made are uncertain or are not supported by robust evidence. An example of both is the assertion in the Harvard

Center on the Developing Child paper *A Science-Based Framework for Early Childhood Policy* that 'the maximal capacity of the immature brain to grow and change means that the early childhood years offer the ideal time to provide experiences that shape healthy brain circuits'.[64]

The footnote to this statement cites three papers – one on primates, one on how the human central nervous system develops in pregnancy and a review of neural development in the first years of life.[65] This review points out that neural development is not limited to the early years: 'To say that infancy and young childhood is the only period in which new neural circuitry is established would grossly understate the complexity of the human neural system.' And, crucially, it highlights how limited our knowledge is: 'The mechanisms of human neural development are still far from being fully understood.'[66]

There is still so much we do not know about the brain. The Santiago Declaration, signed by 136 scientists in 2007, very much holds true today: 'Neuroscientific research, at this stage in its development, does not offer scientific guidelines for policy, practice, or parenting.'[67]

In his fascinating history of how understanding of the brain has evolved over the centuries, Matthew Cobb highlights that despite a 'tsunami of brain-related data being produced by laboratories around the world', we are still very far from having a comprehensive framework of brain function. This is because the brain is 'mind-bogglingly complicated. A brain – any brain, not just the human brain . . . – is the most complex object in the known universe.'

Cobb highlights how little we know about even simple nervous systems like the gastric mill in a lobster's stomach which grinds its food:

Decades of work on the connectome [that is, a map of the wiring] of the few dozen neurons that form the central pattern generator in the lobster stomatogastric system, using electrophysiology, cell biology and extensive computer modelling, have still not fully revealed how its limited functions emerge. That brutal, frustrating fact is the benchmark for all claims about understanding the brain.

Cobb explains that a single theory of brain function may not be possible, not even in a worm, because brains are simultaneously integrated and composite. For instance, sight and smell work differently both computationally and structurally. He argues that this may mean that our future understanding of how the brain works will be fragmented, composed of different explanations for different functions. Cobb concludes, 'It is hard to predict how we will eventually come to understand the brain, and what that understanding will consist of.'[68]

Toxic Stress and Corrosive Cortisol

Neuroscience has a seductive allure but also holds sway because it is difficult for the layperson to interrogate the evidence for brain claims. As the neuroscientist Paul Howard-Jones points out, neuromyths, such as the 'once and for all' nature of the first three years, are able to flourish because the scientific concepts are complex and the evidence behind the claims is either hidden in technical journals or is untestable: 'Protected from scrutiny, a range of emotional, developmental and cultural biases have influenced the types of unscientific ideas that have emerged.'[69]

The concept of toxic stress is a good example of the flimsy evidence being used to make bold claims (recall that this was originally called 'chemicals in the brain' but 'toxic stress' was regarded as more powerful). A widely cited 2005 paper from the National Scientific Council on the Developing Child states:

When children experience toxic stress, their cortisol levels remain elevated for prolonged periods of time. Both animal and human studies show that long-term elevations in cortisol levels can alter the function of a number of neural systems, suppress the immune response, and even change the architecture of regions in the brain that are essential for learning and memory.[70]

These confident claims are based on shaky foundations. Cortisol is a hormone secreted by the adrenal glands just above the kidneys. The argument that it can have a negative impact on the long-term functioning of the hypothalamic–pituitary–adrenal (HPA) axis, which regulates many bodily functions, is a hypothesis. One of the leading researchers on cortisol has called it a 'conceptual model'.[71] It largely derives from animal experiments and studies of maltreated children.

But even this evidence is weak. A 2017 meta-analysis of twenty-seven studies exploring the relationship between maltreatment and cortisol found only a small association between maltreatment and low (not high) wake-up cortisol levels among studies with more rigorous designs. There was no significant relationship between the cortisol awakening response or in the degree of change in cortisol levels throughout the day.[72] A 2022 systematic review and meta-analysis which considered eighty-seven studies in order to explore the relationship between HPA axis functioning and child maltreatment stated that 'a comprehensive conclusion about the functioning of the HPA axis in individuals who have been exposed to child maltreatment cannot be drawn at this time point'.[73]

The animal studies aren't conclusive either. For instance, one study among squirrel monkeys concluded that repeated exposure to early life stressors that are challenging, but not overwhelming, could help foster resilience.[74] Another study subjected newborn male mice to stress by removing them from their mother at irregular and frequent intervals and by severely stressing the mothers as well. They observed that the offspring of the stressed mice showed more behavioural flexibility when set tasks than the control group.[75] But we don't hear these studies being spun to claim that stress is good for the brain.

Cortisol is portrayed as a sort of poison, with emotive references to babies' brains being 'flooded' with it.[76] Darcia Narvaez, a professor of psychology, has claimed that an excess of cortisol is 'a neuron killer'.[77] Even the word 'cortisol' sounds awful, conjuring up a sinister substance which invisibly dissolves brains.

However, cortisol is actually essential for the maintenance of normal bodily functions.[78] I was both amazed and outraged when I learned this, having assumed from what I'd read that cortisol is generally harmful. Waking up in the morning, eating and exercise all cause cortisol levels to rise. It is used as a marker of stress in research because it is often elevated in response to psychosocial stress. There are adverse effects associated with both very high and very low levels of cortisol (too little is potentially life-threatening).

We just don't know what levels of cortisol are potentially problematic. A guide for researchers on using cortisol to measure stress states: 'It is still unclear what has the most significant impact on health: cortisol level, slope, pattern or consistency of pattern.'[79] Cortisol levels can differ significantly between individuals. Complicating factors found in adult measurements are waking time, sleep duration and workday versus weekend status.[80]

Despite all the drawbacks in using cortisol as a measure, it comes up a lot in prescriptions about babies and is used unashamedly to promote particular points of view about child-rearing. The clinical psychologist Oliver James knits together a series of studies about cortisol levels in day care to claim: 'There is now overwhelming evidence that day care causes children to have abnormal cortisol levels, probably increasing the risk of behavioural problems like aggression, fearfulness and hyperactivity.'[81] The evidence is only overwhelming if it is judged by faith rather than logic.

Cortisol is also used to counsel against sleep training. The study usually cited in support of this is full of holes. It measured cortisol levels in twenty-five babies aged between four and ten months of age who were taking part in a five-day inpatient sleep training programme. This involved encouraging the babies to self-settle by being left to cry. On the first day, the mothers' and babies' cortisol levels were positively associated when the babies expressed distress. By day three, the babies were no longer showing distress, but their cortisol levels were still regarded as 'elevated'. The researchers concluded that they had 'high levels of physiological distress' and 'were not learning how to internally manage their experiences of stress and discomfort'.

However, this confident certainty is hard to justify. There was no baseline measure or control group to put the levels of cortisol in context and, as is the case for all research using cortisol as a measure, we don't know whether the levels measured are concerning. And, most obviously of all, the very act of taking the cortisol swab, which was done by a nurse rather than the mother, may have caused levels to rise.[82] But an apparent link between cortisol and sleep training has now been established, and it is another thing for women to worry about. Grace Timothy, in her memoir about new motherhood, recalls fretting about 'the threat of cortisol surges and future mental health issues' when contemplating her baby's sleep.[83]

Sue Gerhardt's book *Why Love Matters: How Affection Shapes a Baby's Brain* has helped to make cortisol a popular bogeyman. The book, published in 2004, has attained canonical status in the UK. It is routinely cited in policy and practice documents and included on reading lists for health visitors and midwives.[84] Gerhardt, like Allan Schore, whose work she draws on heavily, comes from a psychoanalytic background strongly influenced by Freud and Bowlby (more on both in Chapter 5 which explores attachment theory). This is a world view which assumes that early childhood experiences – and in particular mothers – shape later life. Schore's key intellectual contribution was to yoke together neuroscience and attachment theory to make this case, with mothers at the heart of it. He wrote in 1994: 'The child's first relationship, the one with the mother, acts as a template, as it permanently shapes the individual's capacity to enter into all later emotional relationships.'[85]

Gerhardt stresses the dangers of what she describes as 'corrosive cortisol' and claims that 'cortisol can have permanent effects on the developing baby's central nervous system'.[86] Her book paints a terrifying picture of the fragile infant brain. Like the Harvard Center on the Developing Child reports, the book is a mix of animal studies and research on maltreated children and adults, with hypotheses spun into certainties. In the 2014 edition of her book, Gerhardt cites the first Luby study discussed in this chapter (the 'Mom's love good for child's brain' one) along with yet another animal study (mice, not acknowledged of course) and (bafflingly) a study on treatment for depression to justify the claim that 'warm, supportive early mothering . . . *promotes* [original emphasis] neurogenesis [that is, the growth of new neurons in the brain]'.[87]

My antipathy towards Gerhardt's work is deeply personal. I read *Why Love Matters* when my son was five weeks old. It had a profoundly negative impact on me, making me feel like a bad mother who was damaging her son. Like many new mothers, I felt overwhelmed with the responsibility I had for my tiny newborn. I was terrified I would break him or hurt him in some way. These fears expanded into new, more chilling, areas after reading about how babies' brains develop and how 'delicate' their physiological systems are. To give one example, Gerhardt writes of the 'enormous power' of negative looks from mothers. At the time, I was exhausted, teary and could barely raise a smile. I felt like I was failing my baby as a result, damaging his fragile, developing brain in ways I could not see. It took me to the edge of a dark precipice. The support of family and friends, and my son's growing responsiveness, pulled me back.

Later, when I began to understand the flimsy scientific foundations of neuroscience narratives, I became incensed. I remain angry, because brain claims heap guilt upon individual mothers and provide a smokescreen that obscures all the social injustices that blight children's futures.

A (Brain) Picture Is Worth a Thousand Words

Damaged brains are central to neuroscience narratives. Gerhardt, for instance, writes about the brains of Romanian orphans having 'a virtual black hole' where their orbitofrontal cortex should be.

An iconic image which has been, in the words of sociologist Hilary Rose and neuroscientist Steven Rose, 'extensively replicated' shows two contrasting children's brains.[88] One is labelled 'normal', the other 'extreme neglect'. The latter is a smaller image, seemingly shrivelled and with two dark holes. The difference is stark and, as Rose and Rose point out, far more dramatic than the brain scans of severely neglected children rescued from Romanian orphanages in the 1990s.

This image has been used to justify sweeping claims about the early years, particularly the role of mothers. For instance, a *Daily Telegraph* article extravagantly claimed (and note the phrase 'constantly and fully responsive'– nothing less will do):

> The primary cause of the extraordinary difference between the brains of these two three-year-old children is the way they were treated by their mothers. The child with the much more fully developed brain was cherished by its mother, who was constantly and fully responsive to her baby. The child with the shrivelled brain was neglected and abused. That difference in treatment explains why one child's brain develops fully, and the other's does not.[89]

The picture of the normal and shrunken brains appeared in an influential 2008 report *Early Intervention: Good Parents. Great Kids. Better Citizens* which was written by the Conservative MP Iain Duncan Smith and the Labour MP Graham Allen. This report went to town on brain claims: 'Neuroscience can now explain why early conditions are so crucial: effectively, our brains are largely formed by what we experience in early life.'[90]

The picture was promoted to the front cover of two subsequent reports written by Graham Allen which were commissioned by

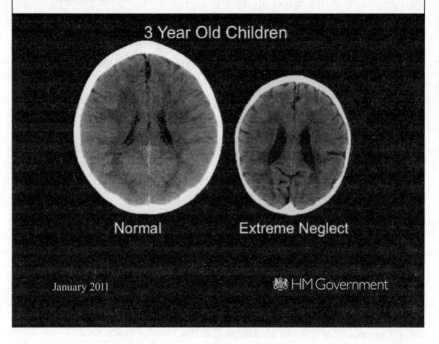

Early Intervention:
The Next Steps

An Independent Report to Her Majesty's Government
Graham Allen MP

3 Year Old Children

Normal   Extreme Neglect

January 2011   HM Government

the UK government.[91] One report cover also included an image of a stack of gold bars to drive home how much money could be saved through early intervention.[92] These reports continued in a similar vein to the first one, recycling the work of the Harvard Center on the Developing Child and Allan Schore, together with a collection of animal studies and research on maltreated children. In a withering critique, the academics David Wastell and Sue White note drily that 'although "journal science" is invoked, he seems not much interested in what it actually says'.[93]

So what do we know about the child with the shrunken brain? The image first appeared in *Brain and Mind*, a short-lived journal, in a paper written by Bruce Perry, an American psychiatrist.[94] Little detail was given about the image beyond the fact that the child had experienced 'severe sensory-deprivation neglect' (that is, minimal exposure to language, touch and social interaction).

Given the significance of the image, neuroscientists and other researchers have tried to find out more. For instance, to what extent was malnutrition also an issue? The role of adequate nutrition in brain development is routinely overlooked in favour of mother blame. Were there any genetic or physiological conditions which may have impacted brain growth? And why was the extreme neglect scan a smaller image than the 'normal' one?[95]

Hilary Rose and Steven Rose wrote to Dr Perry to find out more. He replied that 'due to a variety of factors, we were really unable to conclude much more than "severe neglect impacts brain development"'.[96] Perry later criticised Duncan Smith for claiming that children brought up in abusive or neglected households would grow smaller brains, saying that Duncan Smith had 'greatly misrepresented' and 'distorted' his work. Perry argued it was wrong to apply his work with children who suffered extreme forms of neglect, such as being locked in a basement without human contact, to children who had experienced a far less severe lack of care.[97] But this sleight of hand is typical in neuroscience advocacy. Extrapolating from serious cases of deprivation to ordinary families is a common tactic.

We do not need brain scans to tell us that childhood maltreatment can have many harmful consequences. Researchers have found that abuse and neglect are associated with a range of negative outcomes in adulthood, including poor mental health, drug and alcohol abuse and lower educational achievement.[98] We know from our own experiences, and from books, plays, poems and films, how much adults can damage children.

Neuroscience may one day help us understand how best to prevent maltreated children from developing mental health problems. This is the hope of the psychologists Mattia Gerin, Elly Hanson, Essi Viding and Eamon McCrory. In their review of the evidence, they discuss how childhood maltreatment is associated with alterations in brain function, for instance the processing of threat cues such as angry faces. But there is a long way to go. The review points out that 'there are still common methodological shortcomings that characterise the neuroimaging literature of maltreatment that need to be addressed in future research if stronger causal inferences are to be made'. These include the familiar issues of small sample sizes and conflating severe and less severe maltreatment. There is also much more to learn about the mechanisms at play and what factors may foster resilience.[99]

This painstaking and cautious line of enquiry may come to little – a risk inherent in all scientific endeavour – but it holds out more hope to humanity than alarmist pictures of shrivelled brains.

The Poverty of Brain Claims

There are now many players with a vested interest in using neuroscience to demonstrate the importance of early intervention. The sociologist Jan Macvarish has highlighted the interplay between 'the demand from political actors for legitimising claims and the supply of these claims by a network of advocacy groups, social entrepreneurs, service providers and persuasive individuals'.[100] We shall meet some of these suppliers in later chapters.

Charities and advocacy groups habitually use brain claims to make their case. For instance, a Save the Children report on early learning and child literacy is called *Lighting Up Young Brains: How Parents, Carers and Nurseries Support Children's Brain Development in the First Five Years*. It draws heavily on the work of the National Scientific Council on the Developing Child and even has half a page excitedly explaining different brain scanning techniques.[101]

For some political players, neuroscience has a particularly seductive allure because it provides a new – and apparently scientifically based – justification for laying the responsibility for children's development firmly at the door of parents, particularly mothers. In his report, *Early Intervention: The Next Steps*, the MP Graham Allen breathlessly writes:

> The phenomenal growth of children's brains in the first years of life . . . creates exceptional opportunities, especially for mothers, to provide children with the social and emotional foundations that are the key to personal development and achievement and the best single way to tackle inter-generational dysfunction.[102]

Other factors which impact on children's life chances are pushed out of view. Allen's report mentions poverty only once, when he notes in passing that while most parents want to do their best for their child, factors such as poverty, mental ill health, addiction and violence can make this difficult.

Making parents responsible for resolving societal problems neatly fits a neoliberal agenda which puts the onus on the individual and ignores wider social and economic forces. As Hilary and Steven Rose explain:

> Neuroscience's methodological focus on the individual brain is in accord with that of neoliberalism on the individual rather than the collective . . . In this economy, brains (not the children that surround them) as the repository of mental capital are seen as a resource, and parents are required to lift their children out of poverty by way of their neurons and the magic of brain plasticity.[103]

Incidentally and ironically, in their paper *Science Does Not Speak for Itself*, Shonkoff and Bales said that one of their goals is to get policymakers and the public to understand the impact of factors such as poverty and discrimination on children's development.

The various policy reports on the early years disseminated over the past two decades generally airbrush out inequalities. A UK government report published in 2021 only mentions poverty in passing ('extreme poverty' can be bad for a baby's development if it causes chronic stress – not in and of itself). The report, in the familiar pattern, lifts material from the Harvard Center on the Developing Child reports and tells us that the human brain 'becomes hardwired by the baby's earliest experiences, having a lifelong impact on their physical and emotional health'.[104]

This report is entitled *The Best Start for Life: A Vision for the 1,001 Critical Days* (note the 'best' in the title). The concept of the '1,001 Critical Days' (that is, from pregnancy until the age of two) has been eagerly embraced in the UK, crystallising in the foundation of the First 1001 Days Movement which describes itself as 'an alliance of charities, parliamentarians, academics, and practitioners with a shared passion for babies' emotional wellbeing'.[105]

For this coalition, it is pregnancy and the first two years that really count. In the foreword to *The Best Start for Life*, the Conservative MP Andrea Leadsom writes in urgent tones:

> Two is too late! We spend billions on challenges in society from lack of school readiness to bullying to poor mental health to addictions and criminality; and further billions on conditions such as obesity, diabetes, and congenital heart disease. Yet, the building blocks for lifelong emotional and physical health are laid down in the period from conception to the age of two . . . a strong, supportive policy framework in this area can truly change our society for the better, while saving billions for taxpayers.

In the US, on the other hand, the focus is on the first three years, the period identified as crucial in the 1994 report *Starting Points* we came across earlier which sparked political interest in the infant brain. There is even an advocacy organisation called ZERO TO THREE (its current tagline is 'early connections last a lifetime').[106] Others concentrate on the first five years, like the Save the Children *Lighting Up Young Brains* report mentioned earlier.

This emphasis on the early years disregards what we have learned in the past twenty years about how the brain's structure and functions mature (plasticity, in contrast, is the brain's life-long ability to adapt to changes in its environment). Sarah-Jayne Blakemore is a neuroscientist who has published hundreds of studies on the adolescent brain. She describes how adolescence is a distinct stage in brain development in her fascinating book *Inventing Ourselves: The Secret Life of the Teenage Brain*. Significant changes take place during the teenage years and into the twenties. She explains that until the late 1990s, neuroscience data had suggested that most brain development occurs early in life. This was because research had mostly focused on the auditory and visual areas of the brain in animals, which develop relatively early. Work since then has revealed that different brain regions develop at different rates. As Blakemore says:

> The precise age at which an individual's brain stops developing probably depends on multiple factors, including genetic and environmental influences. Thus it varies from person to person. It might be more useful to consider the age at which brain development ceases as a broad age range rather than a specific number of years. The scientific studies suggest that in most people the brain will have stopped developing by the forties.[107]

Claims about the unique importance of the early years in brain development – whether this be the first two, three or five years – and the opportunities this offers to improve things for children and for society are not based on sound evidence.

In contrast, we have robust data that poverty, and in particular persistent poverty, can disadvantage and harm children. For instance, an analysis of 8,741 children over four waves of the large-scale UK Millennium Cohort Study, which I referred to earlier in this chapter, found that children born into poverty have significantly lower test scores at the ages of three, five and seven. Children at seven persistently living in poverty had substantially lower scores than children who had never experienced poverty. This finding remained robust even after controlling for a wide range of background characteristics and various dimensions of the 'home learning environment' (for example, how often the child is read to or taken to the library).[108]

Later waves of the UK Millennium Cohort Study, which looked at children's physical and mental health at the age of fourteen, found that 'any exposure to poverty was associated with worse physical and mental health outcomes.' For instance, 18% living in poverty throughout their childhood had socioemotional behavioural issues (for example, losing their temper, fighting, being unhappy, nervous or picked on) compared with 6% of children who had never lived in poverty.[109]

'Poverty in early childhood, prolonged poverty, and deep poverty are all associated with worse child and adult outcomes' was the conclusion of the National Academies of Sciences, Engineering, and Medicine in its review of the evidence on child poverty in the US. Children growing up in families below the poverty line are more likely to have worse physical and mental health, lower educational attainment and less employment success compared with children from wealthier families. The evidence suggests that it is poverty in and of itself that disadvantages children; programmes that alleviate poverty have been shown to improve child wellbeing.[110]

All the heat and smoke generated by the various reports and policy documents which reference each other to justify their brain claims obscure how factors such as poverty blight children's life chances. The road of responsibility still leads back to mothers, but mother blame is now wrapped in the mantle of neuroscience.

Magical Thinking

In her account of the rise and fall of the bonding myth, Diane Eyer suggests that magical thinking may have played a role:

> The belief that infants and children are so profoundly shaped by their mothers that a few hours of contact with them could inoculate the babies from harm – even enhance their lives for years to come – would seem to border on magical thinking.[111]

It is as if mothers can cast a spell on their babies, good or bad, that lasts forever. Magical thinking derives from our tendency to find causal relationships where there are none and our difficulty in understanding or accepting the notion of chance. Familiar examples are ceremonial dances to make the rain come or believing that your team lost the match because you forgot to wear your lucky scarf. In his magisterial work charting the decline of magic and rise of religion in sixteenth- and seventeenth-century England, the historian Keith Thomas concludes by arguing that humans will always be prone to magical thinking. This is because it gives us a sense of control over things which feel unpredictable and unmanageable: 'If magic is to be defined as the employment of ineffective techniques to allay anxiety when effective ones are not available, then we must recognise that no society will ever be free from it.'[112]

Magical thinking is very much at work when it comes to the early years. It is used to ward off uncertainty and alleviate our anxieties. It may seem counterintuitive, but scientific and magical thinking are not mutually exclusive. Psychologists Carol Nemeroff and Paul Rozin point out that people can employ multiple modes of thinking with ease, blending 'scientific' with 'magical' approaches.[113] Good Mother myths are justified by science which is more akin to magical thinking.

Returning to the rat study this chapter started with, the press release is infused with magical thinking. It claims that 'erratic maternal care of infants can increase the likelihood of risky behaviours, drug seeking and depression in adolescence and adult life'.[114] Depressed teenagers behaving riskily and taking drugs taps into our deepest fears as parents and as a society. But there is, it is averred, a way to avert these dangers. It is 'crucial' to avoid fragmented and unpredictable care in the baby years. We must therefore turn off our mobile phones to see off the spectre of drugs and depression.

Similarly, early intervention for babies and toddlers is presented as some sort of magic potion by policymakers and politicians. But parenting programmes are not going to level the playing field for disadvantaged children. 'It is magical thinking to expect that if we intervene in the early years, no further help will be needed by children in the elementary school years and beyond,' concluded developmental psychologist Jeanne Brooks-Gunn in her review of evaluations of US early intervention programmes.[115] These later years are also crucial in so many ways. As Sarah-Jayne Blakemore points out, the 'emphasis on early interventions is at odds with the findings that the human brain continues to develop throughout childhood and adolescence and into early adulthood'.[116]

In the same review of early intervention programmes, the developmental psychologist Edward Zigler made an argument which still holds true today:

> Are we sure there is no magic potion that will push poor children into the ranks of the middle-class? Only if the potion contains health care, child care, good housing, sufficient income for every family, child rearing environments free of drugs and violence, support for all parents in their roles, and equal education for all students in all schools.[117]

Risk and the Pregnant Body, a fascinating report written by a cross-disciplinary group of researchers, highlights the role of magical thinking in managing pregnancy risk. The report explains how empirical evidence is overshadowed by rituals and taboo. The lack of empiricism in the burgeoning field of foetal programming research is explored in some detail in historian of science Sarah Richardson's excellent book *The Maternal Imprint: The Contested Science of Maternal-Fetal Effects*.

The background assumption in much of this research is that what women are exposed to during pregnancy determines the health of their children. Many of these studies fail to consider any other factors at all (one paper analysed 274 studies of maternal exposure and found that 78% had not taken into account any other factors).[118] As Richardson notes: 'Unreplicated findings of small effect sizes and tenuous evidence for epigenetic mechanisms . . . are widely embraced as foundations for scientific hypotheses and rapidly translated into advice.'[119]

The advice dispensed off the back of this research resembles a series of taboos. *Risk and the Pregnant Body* explains how inconsequential actions, like a sip of beer or a bite of sushi, are framed as dangerous, likened to poisons which contaminate the pregnant body. By following the rules – and avoiding beer, sushi and all the other things pregnant women are told not to consume, rules which vary from country to country – we can try to ward off the uncertainty and potential perils of pregnancy.[120] The notion that drinking before a baby is even conceived could change the shape of their face, as the study considered in the last chapter claimed, sounds like some grotesque folktale to warn women off behaving badly.

The interplay of science and magic is easier to see with the passage of time. We may scoff now at phrenology, the theory that measuring the contour of the skull can predict personality traits. But it was widely believed in the first half of the nineteenth century, counting both Karl Marx and Queen Victoria among its adherents. Matthew Cobb observes that 'virtually every cultural figure in the nineteenth-century English-speaking world, from Mark Twain to George Eliot, embraced phrenology at one point or another.'[121]

I predict that the notion that mother love can make children's hippocampuses bigger, and solve knotty social problems at the same time, will have a similar fate to phrenology.

Science Really Doesn't Talk

Science is used and abused in the service of various moral and political ends, from warning women off their mobile phones to telling them to interact with their babies in a certain way (more on this in a later chapter). The 'evidence' is used to deflect attention away from problems such as poverty, with extravagant and unfounded claims about how we can make the world a better place through our babies' brains.

The apparent objectivity and truth of science has the effect of shutting down debate. The point Kate Millett made in *Sexual Politics* in 1969 about sociology applies to science more generally: 'Through its pose of objectivity, it gains a special efficacy in reinforcing stereotypes'.[122] The use of science to justify Good Mother myths makes them much harder to challenge.

Science is shaped by human biases and, like fish in water, we are too steeped in some of our beliefs to even notice them. But there is a difference between research that is shaped by cultural assumptions and research which is interpreted and communicated through moral prisms. The former reflects the current status of women in society, while the latter seeks to tell women what they should do and feel. Science should not be used to issue edicts about our behaviour and emotions. Just as it is difficult to 'go against nature', so too is it hard to ignore directives if we think we may end up damaging our children's brains.

'What science tells us' is a common heading in the various papers churned out by the National Scientific Council on the Developing Child. But the use of science in the third person is deeply problematic. It is a fundamental misrepresentation of what science is all about. Science is a method, a means of building and interrogating our knowledge, not a definitive answer.

Science imbued with too much certainty, particularly in areas where we still have much to learn, shades into magical thinking.

It shouldn't need saying, but science is done by people. Scientists can talk, science cannot. And it should stop being used to tell women what to do.

3

Birthing Pains

Science and nature are deployed as separate forms of authority to buttress Good Mother myths, but the prescriptions are generally the same. Birth is different. The twin forces of science and nature are at play, but there are competing credos about whether birth is a natural physiological process or a medical matter requiring the careful management of risk.

In broad terms, the first philosophy is associated with midwives, a 'historically vilified and feted figure' as the historian and midwife Tania McIntosh puts it, the second with obstetricians.[1] The historian Ludmilla Jordanova recounts how eighteenth-century male medical practitioners linked midwives with nature and tradition in their writings, while allying their profession with science and progress. The comparison was intended to attack and undermine – midwives were dangerous and ignorant in contrast with male surgeons and physicians.[2] Using 'nature' as a form of reproach illustrates what a malleable concept it is.

New narratives of birth which challenged masculine medical authority were developed in the second half of the twentieth century. What the literary scholar Tess Cosslett has called 'the "story" of natural childbirth' shifted focus and power from doctors to birthing women.[3] Sheila Kitzinger was an extraordinary woman who was a birth activist, researcher, writer, childbirth educator and a leading light for many years in the National Childbirth Trust. She contended that a medicalised approach to birth mistakenly treats women's bodies as fundamentally flawed. She argued that women in childbirth are 'treated like products on a factory conveyor belt . . . they feel they are not cared for as human beings, but are like "meat on a table", "an oven-trussed turkey" or "fish on a slab". They suffer from institutionalised violence.'[4]

Birth was reclaimed from patriarchal obstetricians and recast, in the words of historian Paula A. Michaels, as a 'fully active, conscious, embodied experience'.[5] Medical management, drugs and other interventions were to be avoided. As Kitzinger put it, with her customary eloquence and passion, 'when a woman has freedom to follow her instincts, and allow the creative force to surge through her, birth-giving can be an act of assent to life, a thanksgiving, and in spite of pain, a sexually intense experience.'[6]

The medical and natural visions of birth compete with each other, leaving women caught in the middle. In their paper *Intuition as Authoritative Knowledge in Midwifery and Homebirth*, the anthropologist Robbie Davis-Floyd and midwife Elizabeth Davis approvingly refer to women 'who supervalue nature and their natural bodies over science and technology'.[7] In the other corner, we have the obstetrician Hans Peter Dietz who has claimed 'natural childbirth ideology is not just dangerous to women and babies, it is becoming dangerous to its adherents.'[8]

Tess Cosslett argues that both discourses prescribe ideals of female behaviour – passivity and obedience in the medical model and joyful, conscious achievement in the natural paradigm. Both visions can be flexed in a number of ways, but because they are in opposition to one another, women can always be found wanting. As Cosslett says: 'The fact that there are *two* dominant, opposing discourses . . . means there will always be at least two kinds of mothers, failing or succeeding according to the two versions.' As we shall see, both discourses are employed to justify judging, shaming and harming women physically and emotionally.

Too Little, Too Late or Too Much, Too Soon?

'Too little, too late' or 'too much, too soon' is how a group of health researchers characterised the under- or over-medicalisation of birth in a *Lancet* paper. In 'too little, too late' scenarios, care is inadequate, unavailable or delayed for too long. 'Too much, too soon' is medicalisation which can cause harm if applied routinely or overused (examples given are continuous electronic foetal monitoring, episiotomies, or enemas on admission for labour).[9]

Whether care is 'too little, too late' or 'too much, too soon' depends on where you are, although they are not mutually exclusive and both can exist in the same setting. The dynamics shaping what happens during birth vary enormously, as evidenced by the wide range of caesarean rates across the world, from less than 1% in South Sudan to 58% in the Dominican Republic.[10] The prevalence of caesareans is not determined by women's bodies or wishes but by resources, power relations and cultural expectations.

In some countries, a dearth of resources in maternity care means that some medical options simply aren't available. Preventable maternal deaths are all too common across the globe. It is estimated that there were 287,000 maternal deaths worldwide in 2020, a rate of 223 deaths per 100,000 live births. These deaths are concentrated in the poorest parts of the world; Sub-Saharan Africa alone accounted for around 70% of global maternal deaths, followed by Central and South Asia on almost 17%.[11] The leading causes of death are haemorrhages, sepsis and hypertensive disorders such as eclampsia. Most of these deaths are avoidable.[12]

In other countries, 'too much, too soon' is more common. The legal scholar Elizabeth Kukura highlights 'the pervasive medicalization of birth' in the US.[13] This has its roots in the victory of the obstetrics profession over midwives and non-specialist doctors, which saw birth rendered as a pathological process requiring medical intervention.

At the turn of the twentieth century, around half of births in the US were attended by midwives, and rates were higher still among Black and immigrant women (86% of all Italian American women giving birth in Chicago according to a 1908 study and 88% of Black mothers in Mississippi according to a 1918 study). But a sustained campaign against midwives by the obstetrics profession, at its height in the period 1910–20, saw numbers steadily drop. Midwives were castigated for being ignorant, dirty, superstitious and even evil, with Black midwives, often known as 'Granny midwives', coming in for particularly venomous criticism. In 1909, 41% of births in New York were attended by midwives, but just over a decade later, in 1920, the figure had dropped to 27%.[14] By 1975, only 0.9% of births in the US were attended by midwives.[15] However, 'Granny midwives' remained common in southern Black communities throughout the 1960s.[16]

One of the strongest critics of midwives was the Chicago physician Joseph B. DeLee, who shaped the field of US obstetrics in the first half of the twentieth century (his textbook *The Principles and Practice of Obstetrics* ran to thirteen editions after first appearing in 1913).[17] DeLee described the midwife as 'a relic of barbarism' who 'destroys obstetric ideals'. These obstetric ideals held that birth is, in DeLee's words, a 'pathologic' process and 'no longer a normal function'.[18] As the historian of medicine Jacqueline Wolf notes, the rise in obstetrics was accompanied by a change in terminology from midwives 'catching babies', which accorded a focal role to the birthing woman, to obstetricians 'delivering' them, which put physicians centre stage.[19]

DeLee believed in a preventative approach to birth, where physicians intervened to avert damage to mothers and babies. He recommended that procedures such as episiotomies (a cut made to the perineum, the tissue between the vagina opening and the anus, to make the vaginal opening wider) should be a routine part of care. In the 1950s, episiotomies were performed in 84% of US births. In the decades that followed, scientific evidence mounted against their routine use, highlighting the likelihood of greater damage to the perineum than a tear. As new narratives of birth started to take hold, activists strongly criticised the routine cutting of women; Sheila Kitzinger described episiotomies as 'ritual mutilation' which meant that 'women start out on motherhood *wounded*'.[20] Their routine use fell out of favour; by 2011 only 9% of births in the US involved an episiotomy.[21]

But maternity care in the US has continued to be pushed in the direction of 'too much, too soon', driven by the profit motive and a fear of litigation. Because of these factors, the caesarean section rate nearly tripled between 1970 and 1978 (from 5.5 to 15.2%).[22] It has continued to climb, reaching 32% in 2007 and staying around that level ever since.[23]

'Technology fetishism in the medical model of birth' is the sociologist Louise Roth's description of the way in which high-tech equipment becomes routine in maternity care. She cites electronic foetal monitoring (EFM), the continuous monitoring of labour contractions and the baby's heartbeat, as a prime example of this. Introduced in 1965, EFM was originally intended for life-threatening situations only. But its use soon became routine, Jacqueline Wolf argues, in part because of media portrayals of 'all births as inherently risky and foetuses as so incessantly threatened that the very process of birth begged for relentless supervision of the foetus'. It was used in 83% of births in 1997, up from 68% in 1989.[24]

Roth highlights the advantages EFM offers hospitals. EFM machines are typically connected to a central nursing station which enables nurses to monitor multiple women at the same time, lowering staff numbers. There is also a marketing element; EFM acts, in Roth's words, as 'a symbol of high-quality, high-tech care'.

But EFM is no more effective in identifying foetal distress than intermittent monitoring using a handheld machine. A Cochrane Review concluded that it has not led to reductions in infant mortality or cerebral palsy. However, it is associated with an increase in caesarean sections and instrumental vaginal births, where a ventouse cap or forceps are used. Part of the reason for this is that EFM has a high false positive rate – in other words false alarms about foetal distress – and interpretation of readings can vary significantly.[25] EFM is not therefore recommended for low-risk labours by the American College of Obstetricians and Gynecologists (ACOG).

Despite this, EFM continues to be pervasive in US maternity care. All the obstetricians and midwives Roth interviewed for her research were aware of ACOG's recommendation and the drawbacks of using EFM. But they all believed that the risk of malpractice litigation and the requirements of insurance companies meant that it had to be used as a matter of course. EFM strips (the print-out of its monitoring records) provide one of the few forms of written documentation available in malpractice cases. Roth observes that health professionals 'believe that they *must* use it to produce paper evidence in the event of a medical malpractice suit, and they feel legally vulnerable if they do not'.

Most obstetricians in the US have experienced at least one malpractice claim (91% according to a 2009 survey of ACOG members), and obstetricians pay higher insurance premiums than other medical specialists. This can have significant financial and emotional impacts for practitioners. One obstetrician told Roth, 'it takes a lot of the joy out of what I do. I think I work three to four months of the year just to pay malpractice insurance.'

Roth concludes that the fear of malpractice lawsuits creates 'a culture of anxiety and risk avoidance. A common strategy for managing risk is to fall back on the medicalization schema: ordering more diagnostic tests and intervening more into labour and birth.'[26] As we shall go on to explore, this does not lead to better maternity care. Although the US spends much more on healthcare than other high-income nations, its rates of infant and maternal mortality are far higher.

Naturally Birthing

In the UK, unlike the US, midwives have remained central to maternity care. At around the time US midwives were being displaced by obstetricians, UK midwives were given legal recognition and professional status through a series of parliamentary acts, starting with the 1902 Midwives' Act. Campaigners such as the Midwives' Institute (which became the Royal College of Midwives in 1947) successfully made the case that professionalising midwifery would help improve infant and maternal mortality. This was despite some doctors invoking familiar tropes that midwives were dirty, ignorant and drunken. The legislation provided for the registration and training of midwives and aimed to gradually eliminate untrained midwives or 'handywomen'. However, handywomen, who were cheaper than midwives and also provided invaluable postnatal support to harried working-class women, continued to play a role in births until the 1940s, when the National Health Service was founded.

Medical models of maternity care took hold in the UK, as well as the US, during the twentieth century. By the 1970s, hospital birth was almost universal.[27] Episiotomies reached their zenith in England in that decade (the rate was 55% in 1977) after midwives were authorised to perform them in 1967.[28]

But financial and cultural dynamics in the UK came to favour vaginal births without medical interventions. Activists such as Sheila Kitzinger and the Association of Radical Midwives, which was founded in 1976, argued that midwives and women were disempowered by medicalisation.[29] Promoting 'normal' birth (that is, no inductions, anaesthesia, instrumental births, or caesareans) has been the orthodoxy for many years. An influential 2007 consensus statement from the Royal College of Midwives, the Royal College of Obstetricians and Gynaecologists, and the National Childbirth Trust successfully lobbied for all NHS trusts to collect statistics on normal births. The aim was to increase the rate of normal births.

Underpinning the consensus statement were the dual assumptions that normal birth is the desire of most women and within their capability:

> With appropriate care and support the majority of healthy women can give birth with a minimum of medical procedures and most women prefer to avoid interventions, provided that their baby is safe and they feel they can cope.[30]

'Normal birth' is probably more commonly known as 'natural birth'. The term 'natural childbirth' was first used by the English obstetrician Grantly Dick-Read, best known for *Childbirth Without Fear: The Principles and Practice of Natural Childbirth*, which was published in 1944. Dick-Read described women as 'adapted primarily for the perfection of womanhood which is, according to the law of Nature, reproduction'. Like others, he invoked the authority of nature to propagate his particular Good Mother myths:

> [Childbirth] means hard work and self-control; it is nature's first lesson in the two greatest assets of good motherhood. Children will always mean hard work and will always demand self-control; this is a small cost price to a right-minded woman.

Dick-Read claimed that in 'more cultured' societies, a woman's fear of childbirth causes muscular tension in the uterus which gives rise to pain. He contrasted this with 'primitive people' who 'accomplished' childbirth 'with comparative ease'. As with attachment theory and breastfeeding advocacy, the 'primitive woman' is a cultural construct, a blank canvas onto which judgements and assumptions can be painted.

Dick-Read's solution to fear in childbirth was educating and training pregnant women so 'they may assist the natural forces and not resist them'.[31] Again we see the paradox that women need to be instructed on things that we are told come naturally to them. Dick-Read's backing of childbirth education is one of the reasons why his advocacy for natural birth has been so influential. He inspired Prunella Briance, whose daughter died during what she described as a 'horribly mismanaged' birth, to found the Natural Childbirth Association in 1956. It was renamed the National Childbirth Trust, or the NCT, in 1961. The NCT has been providing antenatal classes since 1959 (I run NCT postnatal courses, which I believe started in the 1980s).[32]

Dick-Read's theories had some influence in the US, but the French obstetrician Fernand Lamaze became more associated with the natural birth movement there thanks to Marjorie Karmel's 1959 best-seller *Thank You, Dr Lamaze*. Karmel read *Childbirth Without Fear* travelling on a passenger liner from New York to France while pregnant with her first child. The book inspired her to try for a natural birth. Once in Paris, she found Lamaze who had observed the Pavlov method of childbirth being practised in Russian hospitals. Lamaze became an advocate of conditioning women to be relaxed and calm during labour through exercises and education undertaken before birth. In 1960 Karmel and Elisabeth Bing founded the American Society for Psychoprophylaxis in Obstetrics (ASPO), now renamed Lamaze International. Like the NCT in the UK, it continues to provide birth preparation classes.[33]

Dick-Read fought a bitter battle against Lamaze's work, even claiming that his method was a ploy to convert women to communism. His protests were to little avail; his and Lamaze's approaches 'intermingled and hybridised', in the words of Michaels, in the US and the UK. The NCT embraced Lamaze's method of 'prepared' childbirth. In 1958, while his greatest advocate Briance was away in the US, the NCT changed its constitution to remove all mentions of Dick-Read.[34]

Implicit in much natural birth discourse – and to a degree in childbirth education – is the assumption that women can shape what birth they have. This inevitably results in feelings of guilt, blame and failure when things don't go to plan. Eating too much ice cream was one of the reasons why this woman taking part in a Canadian qualitative study blamed herself for having a caesarean section:

> I feel sort of like I failed in the birthing arena . . . maybe if I'd have exercised more or maybe if I'd done something differently maybe I would have been one of those women who pushed. Because that's the ultimate standard . . . I never expected that I'd be someone who had a C-section. Logically I know that it [the C-section] was necessary, but somehow I think, if I was slim and if I had walked every day and not eaten as much ice cream that would not have happened.[35]

Women who do not give birth 'naturally' can feel like they have failed some sort of test of motherhood. This can be exacerbated by the strong undercurrent of moralising which is often found around birth. The good and natural mother 'earns' her babies through a vaginal birth with no pain relief. Women who have caesarean births can be accused of taking the easy option, of being selfish and unwilling to make the sacrifices required of mothers ('too posh to push'). The drugs they receive during child-birth can be portrayed as poisons which contaminate and may even damage the pure baby. Their births are not natural or normal and are therefore unnatural and abnormal.

Beliefs about what women 'naturally' want can result in them being pressurised to take a particular path. Some women involved in a UK qualitative study felt that a 'natural birth' had been pushed upon them during antenatal classes, with 'scaremonger-ing tactics' used to deter them from medicalised options. They felt there had been a lack of realistic information about labour and that their midwives withheld information about interven-tions, leading them to feeling 'anxious, out of control and infantilised'. One woman reflected, 'It's almost like they treat you a bit like a child, like you can't make your own decision so you can't hear anything scary because you won't be able to cope with it.'[36] This can leave women completely unprepared for the possibility of serious birth injuries or other adverse consequences.

We saw both moralism and paternalism at play in a landmark 2015 UK Supreme Court case which recognised women's right to choose their own treatment and to be informed of any risks relevant to them personally. In this case, Nadine Montgomery was not informed that her diabetes meant there was a higher chance of shoulder dystocia, where the baby's shoulder becomes stuck behind the mother's pelvic bone, preventing the birth of the baby's body. Her risk was increased because of her small stature and the size of her baby. When giving evidence, the obstetrician said she did not mention any of this because 'most women will actually say, "I'd rather have a caesarean section" . . . and it's not in the maternal interests for women to have caesarean sections.' Nadine Montgomery's son did indeed experience shoulder dystocia which resulted in brain damage and cerebral palsy. Lady Hale commented in the judgement:

> This does not look like a purely medical judgment. It looks like a judgment that vaginal delivery is in some way morally preferable to a caesarean section: so much so that it justifies depriving the pregnant woman of the information needed for her to make a free choice in the matter.[37]

Nadine Montgomery's case is not the only example of how moral judgements can have grim and tragic consequences for mothers and babies. The Ockenden Review documented two decades of poor care in the Shrewsbury and Telford Hospital NHS Trust. The review estimated that the nine mothers and 201 babies who died could have survived if better care had been provided. There were many factors at play (which we shall come on to), but one important one was a desire to minimise rates of caesareans. One woman said:

> I felt that my concerns during labour were not addressed, that I was made to have a natural birth when an emergency c section

was more appropriate just so they didn't dent their precious natural birth rate target. I felt like I was on a butcher's slab.

The trust's appalling record came to light thanks to the determined campaigning of the parents of Kate Stanton-Davies and Pippa Griffiths. Kate and Pippa's deaths shortly after birth were preventable. Before that point, the trust was praised for having a lower-than-average caesarean section rate. One member of staff said to the Ockenden Review:

> They were always very proud of their low caesarean rates . . . I personally found all the failed/attempted instrumental deliveries very difficult to deal with. I had never seen so many injuries/HIE [damage caused to a baby's brain from lack of oxygen]/resuscitations from this. Nothing to be proud of.[38]

Mistreatment and Coercion

A formidable Good Mother myth is that women should make boundless sacrifices for their children. As we have seen, this belief is used to reproach women who have caesareans, but it can also be deployed against women who don't want medical interventions. Women can be chastised for being self-indulgent for wanting a vaginal birth – or worse still, a birth at home rather than in a hospital – instead of submitting themselves to medicine in the best interests of their baby. Women who want to give birth at home are particularly open to being vilified for doing something risky and dangerous.

Disapproval can shade into coercion, with women forced into medical procedures and unwanted interventions in a variety of ways. It can be physical – being held down, forced into birth positions or tethered to the bed. Some women use the language of sexual assault and rape to describe these experiences. One woman who took part in a study on traumatic birth recalled:

The most terrifying part of the whole ordeal was being held down by four people and my genitals being touched and probed repeatedly without permission and no say in the matter, this is called rape, except when you are giving birth. My daughter's birth was more sexually traumatising than the childhood abuse I'd experienced.

This study was conducted among women from around the world and analysed their responses to the question 'describe the birth trauma experience, and what you found traumatising'. Women related how they were humiliated, belittled and treated like a piece of meat. One woman said:

I felt very bullied, and even violated . . . It was the feeling of disempowerment and not having the right to do with my body what I wished – and that someone else could force me to do something against my will.

As we have explored, invoking harm to a woman's child can be a particularly effective way to coerce her. In the traumatic birth study, women described how their care providers used what some termed the 'dead baby threat' to bully them into accepting interventions or treatment they did not want. Some felt they were lied to about the risks to their baby. One woman disclosed:

I was basically told that if I didn't have a C-section on their timetable I would kill my baby, even though they couldn't tell me what exactly was 'wrong' as to why I was not delivering vaginally . . . They broke me down gradually until they declared my baby was 'in distress' (she wasn't . . . I could see the screens).[39]

In the most extreme circumstances, women are threatened with unmothering to force them to accept unwanted interventions. Elizabeth Kukura recounts two chilling cases. In one, a woman from Virginia was threatened with a court order and being reported to child welfare services if she did not agree to a caesarean. She relented, but the hospital contacted the authorities anyway and removed her baby from her at birth. After three months of interviews and home observations, the agency decided there were no grounds for investigation and closed the case.

In another case, a woman from New Jersey was reported to family services for child neglect and abuse because she refused to consent to a caesarean on the grounds that there was no medical indication that this was necessary. She had a vaginal birth and her baby was healthy. Nevertheless, her newborn baby was put into foster care and her parental rights were terminated.[40]

The issue of consent was explored in a survey conducted by Birthrights, a UK charity which endeavours to improve experiences of pregnancy and childbirth by promoting respect for human rights. Its *Dignity in Childbirth* study among 977 women who had given birth in the past two years found that 12% said that they had not given their consent to examinations or procedures.[41] This can be more subtle than outright coercion. Women may not be properly consulted or made to feel they cannot ask questions or do not have a say. Phrases such as 'we have to . . .' or 'we are going to . . .' assume that the woman is not the one making the decisions.

Vaginal examinations during labour are a good example of a procedure that can happen without women's consent. These examinations are a way of checking how labour is progressing by seeing how far the cervix has dilated. However, as a recent Cochrane Review found, there is no robust evidence that routine vaginal examinations are actually effective in assessing how labour is progressing.[42]

For some women, vaginal examinations can be helpful and reassuring. But for others, they can be distressing and painful (the Ockenden Review heard examples of 'excessive and painful' vaginal examinations). In the traumatic birth study, some women described how they begged and screamed at their care providers to try to get them to stop vaginal examinations. One said, 'The doctor would not get her fingers out of my vagina even when directly told.' Another recounted how her obstetrician assaulted her to get her to agree to having her waters broken:

> She said she wanted to do one more cervical check. I consented and when she did it, she grabbed my cervix and pinched it. She would not let go until I consented to letting her break my water. I was in tears from the pain, screaming, begging and sobbing for her to let go and get her hand out of my vagina. She would not let go until I consented, which I finally did.[43]

The writer Emma Jane Unsworth believes a rough and unwanted vaginal examination may have been a factor in her developing postnatal depression:

> She said she'd examine me. She spoke to me so disrespectfully, I was almost in tears before her fingers were inside. I was assaulted by a boy on the top deck of a bus when I was thirteen and this felt similar. Her fingers rough and mean; her own agenda to fulfil . . . I lost all rights to my body in that moment. I lost all autonomy. I didn't know I could say no. I didn't know I could ask for better . . . I wonder how much of this rage, this disappointment, contributed towards the PND. How much I had to bed it down inside me and push, push, push, down instead of out – until it was a roiling mass in my guts, waiting to blow.[44]

Episiotomies are another procedure that women can be subjected to without their agreement. Only 41% who underwent an episiotomy had been given a choice according to a US study of 2,400 women who had recently given birth.[45] And this figure may be an undercount. A study among women giving birth in Ghana, Guinea, Myanmar and Nigeria explored birth experiences using both surveys (with 2,672 women) and continuous observations of labour and childbirth (there were 2,016 observations). In the survey, 56% of women who had episiotomies said they did not consent, but the figure was even higher in the observations at 75%.[46]

Verbal abuse, where women are shouted at, scolded or mocked, can be a common type of mistreatment during childbirth. The Ghana, Guinea, Myanmar and Nigeria study found that verbal abuse was the most common form of mistreatment observed, seen in 38% of births. This abuse is rooted in power dynamics and attitudes towards women, or particular groups of women. The language used can be degrading, intimidating and infantilising (being called a 'good girl' or told off like a school child) and rob women of their agency and autonomy. Verbal abuse can traumatise women and care becomes unsafe if women are not listened to or are put off speaking up.

Marginalised women are particularly likely to experience verbal abuse and other forms of mistreatment. The US study *Giving Voice to Mothers* found that 17% of the 2,138 women who took part in the research experienced one or more types of mistreatment during childbirth. The most common experiences were being shouted at or scolded by a healthcare provider (9%) and failing to respond to requests for help (8%). Black, Hispanic and Indigenous women were significantly more likely to report mistreatment, compared with White women. Lower socio-economic status was also associated with a higher likelihood of mistreatment.[47]

Verbal abuse can involve belittling women's pain. This was a feature of the abysmal care uncovered by the Ockenden Review. A woman whose baby was on the neonatal unit was criticised for worrying about her pain too much. She was told: 'what we tend to find is that those women who have babies next to them have more important things to think about. People like you who do not, are only concerned with themselves.' Good Mother myths are hard at work here. Another woman who had had surgery after birth to remove a haematoma (a swelling of clotted blood which is potentially life threatening) recounted how she was 'shouted at, ordered about and forgotten . . . I was made to feel like an inadequate mother and made to feel like I was making up how poorly I was and . . . I shouldn't have rung the bell or asked for help'.

The experiences of tennis legend Serena Williams illustrate why not listening to women can end in tragedy. Her story also helps explain racial disparities in maternity deaths. In America, Black women are almost three times as likely as White women to die while pregnant or within one year of the end of a pregnancy. In 2021, the ratio of deaths per 100,000 live births was 26.6 for White women, 28 for Hispanic women and 69.9 for Black women. Rates have increased for all ethnicities, but Black women have seen a particularly sharp rise, almost doubling from 37.3 in 2018 to 69.9 in 2021.[48] In the UK, there is nearly a four-fold difference in maternal mortality rates among Black women and an almost two-fold difference among women from Asian ethnic backgrounds, compared with White women.[49]

Serena Williams was not listened to even though she has a profound understanding of her body. As she says, 'I've suffered every injury imaginable, and I know my body.' She was aware that she was at a high risk of blood clots but was initially ignored when she requested a scan of her lungs and a drip of the drug heparin which helps prevent clots. Despite being in excruciating pain, unable to move and repeatedly coughing, the nurse advised her to rest, telling her, 'I think all this medicine is making you talk crazy.' Williams 'fought hard' and got her scan which showed, as she suspected, a blood clot in her lungs. She reflected:

> Being heard and appropriately treated was the difference between life or death for me; I know those statistics would be different if the medical establishment listened to every Black woman's experience.[50]

The Role of Racism in Mistreatment

Racism can lead to mistreatment during birth because care providers' capacity to see or hear the individual woman is clouded by stereotypes and assumptions. An example is the persistent fiction that Black people feel less pain. We see evidence of this in a US online study among 92 White laypeople and 222 medical students and residents from a university. A majority of both groups (73% and 50%, respectively) endorsed at least one of eleven false beliefs about biological differences between Blacks and Whites, such as 'Blacks' nerve endings are less sensitive than Whites' and 'Black couples are significantly more fertile than White couples'. Students and residents who endorsed more of these beliefs were more likely to think that a Black patient in a mock medical case would feel less pain compared with a White patient.[51]

These beliefs have their roots in slavery and scientific racism. Such stereotypes dehumanise and pathologise Black people as less human. *Systemic Racism, Not Broken Bodies*, Birthrights' inquiry into racial injustice in the UK maternity system, highlights that beliefs that Black bodies are stronger and able to endure more pain coexist with contradictory views about Black and Brown bodies being defective. The inquiry heard testimony about people being deemed higher risk on the basis of their ethnicity and subjected to more surveillance during pregnancy and birth.[52] It also heard multiple examples of the 'strong Black woman' trope. This was something the writer Candice Brathwaite experienced, part of a pattern of bad treatment which left her hospitalised for weeks because an untreated, infected caesarean wound resulted in septic shock. She wrote, 'I had not been cared for, let alone listened to . . . There was this general expectation – even from healthcare providers who looked like me – for me to be strong and silent, or grin and bear it.'[53]

Asian women are stereotyped in different ways, caricatured as being less able to tolerate pain than other women and having a tendency to be too demanding and 'make a fuss about nothing'. The Birthrights inquiry heard from many Asian women who had been subjected to the 'princess' stereotype, for instance being characterised as 'precious'. Black women, on the other hand, were branded as 'aggressive' or 'angry'.

The Birthrights inquiry also heard many examples of incorrect and stereotypical judgements being made, such as assuming Black women are single mothers, Muslim women have lots of children and hijab-wearing women can't speak English. One woman recounted, 'I wore my hijab and abaya during my stay at hospital. Staff in the special care unit were very patronising [until] I disclosed that I was a pharmacist, [when] the whole team's behaviour changed.'

Obstetric Violence

The wide and depressing catalogue of mistreatment of women during childbirth has been officially acknowledged. In 2014, the World Health Organization formally recognised that abuse, neglect or disrespect during childbirth can violate fundamental human rights.[54]

Some activists and scholars have argued that mistreatment during childbirth should be characterised as a form of violence. The term obstetric violence (or 'violencia obstétricia') originates from activism in South America in the 1990s and 2000s which sought to humanise maternity care in settings where over-medicalisation was the norm. Venezuela passed laws prohibiting obstetric violence in 2007, and Argentina, Bolivia, Mexico and Panama later followed suit. The definition in Mexican law explicitly recognises the harm that can be done both by too much (acts) and too little (omissions).[55]

Public health scholars Rachel Jewkes and Loveday Penn-Kekana argue that there are two different dimensions of obstetric violence – the intentional use of violence and structural disrespect. Intentional obstetric violence includes physical and verbal abuse and deliberate withholding of care. Structural disrespect includes unnecessary interventions and lack of staffing and resources. I agree with them that this distinction is necessary to enable 'work on overall improvement in practices whilst holding individuals accountable for more severely abusive actions'.[56]

The concept of obstetric violence derives its power, as Jewkes and Penn-Kekana observe, from the parallels between the mistreatment of women in childbirth and violence against women more generally. Other forms of oppression also need to be recognised. The academic and activist Dána-Ain Davis proposes the term 'obstetric racism', arguing that obstetric violence 'does not adequately take into account the contours of racism that materialize during Black women's medical encounters'.[57] Sociologist Rachelle Chadwick rightly turns our attention to all birthing people. She characterises obstetric violence as a form of violence 'directed at reproductive subjects more broadly (i.e. including trans men, non-binary persons, and those who do not identify as "mothers" or "women")'.[58]

We must recognise the different dimensions of obstetric violence, while also appreciating its deeply gendered nature. Misogyny makes violence against women acceptable and can leave women feeling a deep sense of shame for what they have been subjected to. Kukura observes that cultural expectations of maternal sacrifice can be internalised by women, leading to them 'downplaying the extent of their physical and emotional injuries and choosing not to voice concerns about mistreatment for fear of appearing ungrateful'. This is yet another way in which Good Mother myths can damage women.

Birth Can Damage Bodies

Poor maternal care can leave women with ongoing pain and injuries following childbirth. The list of common injuries is eye-watering: tears or surgical cuts to the perineum, nerve damage, pelvic floor injury and pelvic organ prolapse (where the organs inside the pelvis slip down towards the vagina).

These injuries can result in severe and ongoing physical and psychological difficulties. Most of the 801 women who responded to a survey conducted by three birth trauma charities said birth injuries had impacted on their mental health (85%), their ability to be physically active (74%), their relationship with their partner (65%) and their sex life (83%). Many reported feelings of fear, anxiety and embarrassment. One woman said:

> Although the injury was physical, the psychological impact has been significant. I felt broken and out of control. I feared going to the toilet, going out in public (in case of an accident) and was anxious that having a baby had changed me forever (not in the way I expected). I was so worried that I would never be able to hold my bowel or return to work or walk normally.

Birth injuries can be life-changing. One woman taking part in the survey said: 'Once some of the shock had passed and day to day life went on, I realised how very different my life was going to be going forward. I'm fearful of everything, from sex to exercise.' Another recounted:

> I'm permanently disabled now – something I never thought would happen from giving birth. Not a day has gone past where I haven't been in pain and I don't feel I have my independence anymore . . . I don't hold excitement for myself anymore. I'm scared of my future and what it holds for me.[59]

Urinary or faecal incontinence because of birth injuries can lead to significant practical and emotional difficulties. Women can become trapped at home. One woman taking part in the study said, 'I used to be outgoing, now I prefer to stay home. It's really isolating but I'd rather have an accident at home than [risk] having an accident in public.' There can be feelings of disgust and self-hatred. One woman said: 'I leak urine constantly. I hate myself and my body, I feel disgusting with what has happened to me.'

Women with severe perinatal trauma (that is, tears which reach to the anal sphincter or rectum) reported feeling humiliated by incontinence in a qualitative Australian study exploring the experience of living with these injuries. One woman said:

Like when you're a kid if you pooh your pants, there's this kind of stigma that you're dirty and lazy. And even when you're an adult every time it happened I was just like – oh this is filthy, I'm in my twenties and I can't control myself. I didn't want to talk to anybody about it, I didn't even want to talk to the doctor about it.[60]

When women do talk about their pain, they have no guarantee they will be heard. Caroline Criado Perez has persuasively argued that 'failing to listen to female expressions of pain runs deep'. She documents how 'women's physical pain is far more likely to be dismissed as "emotional" or "psychosomatic".'[61] And when it comes to childbirth, women are simply expected to suck it up. The birth injuries study found that women were often told that their symptoms were normal:

I felt inadequate, silly and totally dismissed. I felt like the doctors wanted me to go away and not cause a fuss and were trying to convince me that what happened to me was normal. In my GP's exact words 'it happens' with a shoulder shrug.

The Ockenden Review also heard instances of women not being listened to about their birth injuries. One woman explained to a consultant that she was passing gas through her vagina. She was told she had a 'baggy fanny' caused by having a large baby and that no further investigation was required. Her injury worsened, resulting in a fistula (an abnormal channel between the vagina and rectum) and passing faeces through her vagina. This was something she had to live with for some time which left her feeling depressed, isolated and blaming herself. She told the Ockenden Review:

Feeling that I should have pushed this matter further in the hospital made me feel inadequate as a mother. With the fistula causing personal care issues for me, the depression got worse. It wasn't diagnosed for quite some time. The emotional effects of all this still affect me 10 years on.

If women's birth injuries are ignored or dismissed, the long-term consequences can be devastating, as this post on Mumsnet illustrates:

I had a stitched up tear that didn't get looked at by the GP at my six week check. Months later it turned out I had retained placenta and needed vaginal reconstruction as a result of very badly done stitches. I got an infection from the second operation and was fobbed off for weeks by the consultant who did the op who didn't believe I was suffering with more than unusual post-op pain. The whole thing was just awful and I can't see myself ever getting over it enough to feel strong enough for a second baby. I am damaged and traumatised for life.[62]

The Trauma of Birth

Feeling traumatised after birth is a depressingly common experience. It has been estimated that one in six (17%) women experience post-traumatic stress symptoms in response to their birth experience and that 4% meet the clinical threshold of post-traumatic stress disorder (PTSD).[63] PTSD symptoms include re-experiencing (for example, flashbacks, nightmares and intrusive memories), avoidance (steering clear of people and situations that remind the sufferer of the traumatic event), hyperarousal (for instance, hypervigilance for threats, irritability, difficulty concentrating and sleep problems) and emotional numbing (blunted feelings, feeling detached from other people and not being able to remember significant parts of the traumatic experience).[64]

Birth trauma can have a profound impact on women's lives. In a brilliant piece of analysis, nursing academic Cheryl Beck mined from her research data the images and metaphors women with PTSD used to describe their experiences. The impact of trauma was often expressed in physical terms; women talked of being surrounded in darkness, drowning at sea, being in a bottomless abyss, feeling like a ticking timebomb and suffocating in layers of trauma. Some women were haunted by constant replays of their trauma. One said: 'After the baby's first night feed, I could never get back to sleep because the birth kept playing in my head like a video on automatic replay.'[65]

There is not a great deal of research on how long birth-related PTSD lasts and how many women recover spontaneously over time. A Turkish study found that forty-two of the seventy-three women who had PTSD at four to six weeks after their deliveries no longer met the criteria at six months, but thirty-one of the women did.[66] However, it is clear from women's accounts that birth trauma can last for many years. One woman commented on a Mumsnet thread that she was still experiencing flashbacks forty-two years after her traumatic birth.[67]

Women are more likely to suffer from PTSD if they have experienced an emergency caesarean section or birth complications. However, studies show that a significant proportion of women with postnatal PTSD symptoms have had seemingly straightforward vaginal births.[68] A negative subjective experience of childbirth has been found to be the most important birth-related predictor for developing PTSD or PTSD symptoms.[69]

As with physical pain, women's experiences of trauma can be minimised. 'At least you have a healthy baby' can be a common rejoinder to women's accounts of difficult births. One woman taking part in the birth injuries study said:

I felt like I failed as a woman as I wasn't able to give birth naturally. I suffered with PTSD and required therapy when pregnant with my second. Friends took away my right to feel traumatised by saying 'at least you've got a healthy baby'.[70]

Kim Thomas, the CEO of the charity Birth Trauma Association, argues that much birth trauma can be avoided. It is important to provide support to women at particular risk because of previous traumatic experiences such as violence, abuse or rape.[71] Minimising the risk of birth trauma is also about providing good care in childbirth for all women and birthing people.

Respectful, Honest and Non-judgemental Care

Safe and respectful care are indivisible. If the focus is simply on safety, women will continue being railroaded and injured and traumatised on the basis that a healthy baby is all that matters. It should go without saying that women and birthing people matter too.

Respectful care means listening to women, understanding them, seeing them as people. Moral judgements and mother blaming should be cast aside. It is wrong to assume that all women want a 'normal birth' and that a desire for medical interventions means they are uninformed. The doula and community health activist Yania Escobar reflects, 'I feel like a lot of the training as a doula focuses on talking people out of getting epidurals, using labour-augmenting drugs, or getting a caesarean section.' She rightly argues, 'If there are medical interventions available people should feel completely legitimized in having them. If somebody wants to get an epidural then they want to get an epidural!'[72] Women should not have information about the potential risks of vaginal birth withheld because they might make different decisions – so what if they do?

There are many good reasons why a woman might want to have a caesarean. Birthrights analysed enquiries from eighty-three women who got in touch with its advice service about maternal request caesareans. The most common reason for asking for a caesarean was a previous traumatic birth, followed by an underlying medical condition, such as fibroids, which did not meet the medical threshold for requiring a caesarean but was causing great anxiety. Other reasons were a fear of childbirth or previous experiences of trauma, such as sexual assault. Birthrights found that even though women in the UK have a right to request a caesarean, many of the health trusts which responded to their freedom of information request only allowed them with conditions, such as requiring permission from two consultants or undergoing a compulsory mental health appointment (with the obvious implication that wanting a caesarean suggests some sort of mental illness). Some trusts simply said an outright 'no' – 15% did not offer maternal request caesareans at all.[73]

Equally, we need to recognise how important vaginal birth without interventions is to some women, what is required to maximise the chances of this happening and how vaginal births can be hindered by hospital care. As the birth worker Kelly Gray explains, try going for a poo with someone poking your rectum while your family watches.[74] Sheila Kitzinger uses a more romantic analogy: 'If we were forced to make love in public, and in the setting of the standard hospital delivery room, we would probably feel inhibited.'[75] Pain relief strategies such as moving around or being in water are not possible where electronic foetal monitoring (EFM) is being used. Women are immobilised by measuring devices secured to the abdomen with elastic belts. If they move around too much, the machine's alarm goes off because the foetal heart rate has been lost.

Birth positions are a good example of the cultural and practical obstacles that can hamper the physiology of birth. The anthropologist Wenda Trevathan's survey of birthing positions in 159 societies found that sitting, kneeling and squatting were the most common (Trevathan also notes that ethnographic reports of birth mention episiotomies, manual dilation of the cervix, herbal medicines and inducing vomiting – interventions during birth are not only found in industrialised societies).[76] A Cochrane Review summarised the advantages of giving birth in upright positions such as sitting, kneeling and squatting: 'The pelvis is able to expand as the baby moves down; gravity may also be helpful and the baby may benefit because the weight of the uterus will not be pressing down on the mother's major blood vessels which supply oxygen and nutrition to the baby.'[77]

When women are filmed giving birth, they are invariably on their backs. An analysis of 123 births depicted in eighty-five US reality-based TV shows found that in 85% of cases women were shown pushing on their backs. Women were also often infantilised (called a 'good girl' during pushing) or discouraged from vocalising. In one example, a physician said, 'Let's have a baby in a nice *civilized* way. No screaming. No yelling.'[78] Similarly in the UK, an analysis of two seasons of the popular long-running TV show *One Born Every Minute* found that 90% of women pushing or having assistance before a baby is born were depicted on their backs.[79]

Women need care providers with the skills, confidence and time to support their labour. So many things can undermine a birthing person and make them feel vulnerable: internal examinations, being left alone, phrases such as 'failure to progress', the beeps of an EFM machine, pronouncements that they are not in labour or being told to labour on their back. And blame and guilt are always waiting in the wings.

With birth, there are the same tensions as breastfeeding, which we will be looking at in the next chapter. Women need to feel confident that their bodies can birth vaginally if this is what they want, but this risks instilling a huge sense of failure if things don't go to plan. The quandary is arguably even more acute than for breastfeeding – the baby (or babies) must get out of a woman's body somehow. Events can unfold very quickly.

I therefore feel ambivalent about how far we should be advocating for vaginal births without medical interventions. The argument that birth is a physiological process does have strong emotional appeal to me personally. One of my births was like this and it was wonderful. My other birth was long, exhausting and ended with a forceps delivery (I narrowly avoided a caesarean). I was adamantly against the idea of a caesarean because I am very squeamish and could not bear the thought of having my abdomen cut. But I was – and to a degree remain – strongly influenced by cultural ideals of birth in the UK.

I also feel some ambivalence about the NCT's role in all of this. I have been a postnatal practitioner with the NCT for more than a decade and have seen firsthand the many different ways in which it can and does support parents. In my experience, its practitioners, staff and volunteers have a strong and sincere commitment to people having good experiences of pregnancy, birth and early parenthood. The NCT has a long tradition of research and providing evidence-based information. It also has a distinguished campaigning record, for example its recent Hidden Half campaign which has shone a light on postnatal mental illness and advocated for better care.

However, the NCT has promoted 'natural' and 'normal' birth for much of its history. This has contributed to a culture where women can be left feeling like failures because their births did not pan out this way. I know that many in the NCT have been acutely aware of this issue and for some years it has taken a more impartial stance in its antenatal classes and content for parents. It expunged the words 'natural birth' from its website around the time the Ockenden Review was published.[80] But some women can still feel guilt-tripped. The writer Eliane Glaser argues that NCT antenatal classes purport to be non-prescriptive but subtly promote 'natural birth' by 'gently' encouraging women to give birth without interventions. She and her antenatal class ended up feeling tricked and traumatised.[81]

It is important to say that this is certainly not everyone's experience. At the time of writing, the NCT is not publishing its course evaluations, but all the data I have seen over the years shows that a large majority rate their antenatal course as good or excellent. The journalist Rebecca Holman described her NCT course leader as 'really pragmatic, non-judgmental . . . open to discussing and answering questions on all forms of childbirth, pain relief and feeding'.[82]

A practical, honest and non-judgemental approach is the way to resolve the conflict between science and nature. We should not make assumptions about what women want or moralise about what they should or should not do. Honesty is key. Many women are able to birth vaginally – with or without medical interventions – but there are no guarantees and countless things can get in the way of this. There are no guarantees about caesarean births either; the course of recovery can vary enormously. Birth is an unpredictable business, and there is a limit to how much we can control.

We Need Systemic Change

The Black Mamas Matter Alliance has proposed a new care model for Black women in *Setting the Standard for Holistic Care of and for Black Women*. At the heart of this is seeing a Black woman as a person:

> When working with Black women patients, it is essential that providers and staff adopt a lens to see more than the racialized stereotypes associated with the patient in front of them. Seeing Black women as whole, educated, loved, valued, and valuable is essential to good care. Black women deserve high quality care and must be treated as such.[83]

An LGBT Foundation report makes similar recommendations for maternity care for trans and non-binary people. Its research among eighty-five trans and non-binary birth parents found that 'not being afforded the appropriate agency, dignity, and respect are particular barriers to trans and non-binary birthing parents feeling safe and comfortable accessing services'. The report recommends 'holistic and personalised care' in the form of a personalised care support plan.[84]

These policies are vital, but they are not enough on their own, as the state of maternity care in the UK illustrates. Personalised maternity care grounded in choice has been a central plank of health policy since the landmark 1993 report *Changing Childbirth* was published by the Department of Health. National clinical guidelines issued in 2014 recommended 'a culture of respect for each woman as an individual undergoing a significant and emotionally intense life experience, so that the woman is in control, is listened to and is cared for with compassion, and that appropriate informed consent is sought'.[85]

As we have seen, the reality can fall far short of this. The Ockenden Review was not the first investigation into dangerous maternity care in the UK. A 2015 report on the Morecambe Bay NHS Trust found a 'lethal mix' of clinical incompetence, poor working relationships, the pursuit of normal childbirth 'at any cost' and repeated failures to properly investigate or learn from adverse incidents. This resulted in the unnecessary deaths of one mother and eleven babies.[86]

The Ockenden Review found that all of these factors were at play in Shrewsbury and Telford as well – the lessons of Morecambe Bay were not learned. There have also been serious failings in maternity care in Nottingham and East Kent resulting in independent reviews (led by Donna Ockenden again in the case of Nottingham).

As well as the human cost of dangerous maternity care, there is a high financial price. In 2022–3, NHS England paid out £2.6 billion in clinical negligence payments. Not far off half of this amount, 41%, related to maternity care, which meant that around £1.1 billion that could have been spent on healthcare was used to compensate families for avoidable deaths and injuries.[87]

Systemic change is therefore required. We need to recognise where the power is in maternity care and how this can particularly disadvantage marginalised women. Current power dynamics enable women to be mistreated, coerced, dehumanised and silenced. The Birthrights inquiry into racial injustice in maternity care highlights the need to create safe and inclusive workforce cultures. Black and Brown women and birthing people – all women and birthing people – should be decision-makers in their care and in the wider maternity system.[88]

In the US, the model of maternity care is broken. As we have seen, maternal mortality is rising, which is bucking the global trend of falling maternal mortality rates.[89] This is despite the US spending much more on health than other high-income countries. The US devotes 18% of its GDP to healthcare, compared with an average of 10% among the thirty-eight countries that make up the Organisation for Economic Co-operation and Development (OECD). The next biggest spender is Germany on 13% (the UK is not that far behind on 12%). This translates into an average health spend per person of $11,912 in the US, compared with $7,382 in Germany (again the next highest) and $5,388 in the UK.

Despite this greater health spend, the US has considerably higher rates of maternal deaths. The rate is 23.8 per 100,000 live births in 2020, well above the OECD average of 9.8, and far outstripping the Netherlands, the best performing country on 1.2 (the UK's rate is 6.5). We see the same pattern for infant mortality. The rate in the US is 5.4 deaths per 1,000 live births, compared with an OECD average of 4.1. Norway has the lowest rate of all (1.6), while the UK is on 3.6.[90] As with maternal deaths, there is the same pattern of racial disparities. This is regardless of income; an analysis of Californian birth records between 2007 and 2016 found that infant mortality for Black infants in the top tenth of the income distribution is higher than among White infants in the bottom tenth (4.3 deaths per 1,000 births for Black babies, compared with 3.5 for White babies).[91]

The Black Mamas Matter Alliance advocates replacing existing 'hierarchical, rushed, and profit-centred models of care' with alternative models which are already found in communities of colour. These are rooted in partnerships between women, healthcare providers and paraprofessionals such as doulas.[92] The proportion of births attended by midwives in the US is slowly creeping up, rising from 0.9% in 1975, to 6% in 1996, 10% in 2016 and then 12% in 2021.[93] But access to midwives is limited and varies widely geographically, with only 1% of births in Arkansas being attended by midwives compared with 32% in Alaska. State regulations and insurance companies shape the availability of care (a 2014 survey found that 47% of insurance companies did not cover birth centres).[94]

The alternative to the current patchwork of maternity provision in the US is universal healthcare which enables everyone to access high-quality maternity services. Louise Roth argues that universal health insurance, together with public funds to compensate victims of medical errors, would reduce the threat and impact of lawsuits. US malpractice awards relating to childbirth are higher than in the UK, Australia and Canada because of the lack of publicly funded resources for people with lifelong and significant disabilities. As Roth notes: 'The US has the highest litigation rates in the world, as well as the only private, for-profit health insurance system in the developed world – and that is no coincidence.'[95]

Essential to any model of care is ensuring that women and birthing people are looked after by people they can trust and who understand their needs and wishes. Carers need to explain the different options – and what is happening before and during birth – in an honest, clear and respectful way. All forms of birth carry some risk, but how these risks are weighed is shaped by who you are and what matters to you. However women want to birth, they should be treated with care and respect and be central to decision-making.

This is harder to achieve if care providers don't meet someone until they are in labour. A Cochrane Review assessed the impact of midwife continuity models which provide care from the same midwife or team of midwives during pregnancy, birth and the early parenting period, with other care providers involved if required. The review found a lower risk of instrumental births and episiotomies and a greater likelihood of a positive birth experience. It also found some evidence of a cost-saving effect compared with other care models.[96] There is evidence from two UK studies and a US study that continuity of care can be beneficial for marginalised women and result in fewer babies being born prematurely or with low birth weights.[97] Both are important markers of public health because they are associated with a higher risk of mortality and health problems in childhood and adulthood.[98]

Properly resourced maternity care is essential to making birth better for everyone. Inadequate resources are a key factor in mistreatment and poor – even dangerous – maternal care. Some researchers have linked obstetric violence to difficult working conditions. A literature review on obstetric violence observed that the work environment can be precarious and stressful due to limited resources, long shifts and inadequate staff levels.[99] As Rachelle Chadwick says, 'health care providers are themselves potential victims of broader structural disrespect and obstetric violence (e.g., their work is not valued, they are themselves often subject to bullying, and toxic work conditions)'.[100]

There is not a great deal of research on this, but health workers can experience trauma too. A survey among 1,095 members of the Royal College of Obstetricians and Gynaecologists found that 18% of consultants and trainees reported clinically significant PTSD symptoms.[101] In a US study of 464 labour and delivery nurses, 35% reported moderate to severe levels of secondary traumatic stress. In describing their experiences, nurses used phrases such as 'felt like an accomplice to a crime' or 'the physician violated her'.[102]

Birth matters. Women and birthing people should be valued, so too should people who work in maternity care. Structural disrespect harms everyone. Maternity and postnatal care should be properly resourced. Women need to be looked after following birth: I have heard many horror stories over the years of women being left alone and in pain and being subjected to an array of humiliations and privations.

There must be speedy diagnosis and treatment of birth injuries. It should never be OK for women to continue to be in pain. The UK's National Institute for Health and Care Excellence has observed that persistent perineal pain can occur in up to 10% of women one year after vaginal childbirth and describes this as 'a largely neglected area of need'.[103] This is both unsurprising and unacceptable.

Mental health in the perinatal period must also be prioritised; suicide is the leading cause of death in the period between six weeks and one year after birth in the UK and is a leading cause of mortality in the US during pregnancy and for the first year after birth.[104] There should be a focus on both the prevention and treatment of mental health problems. Specifically on birth trauma, while the aim should be to stop it from happening at all, if women do experience it, this should be recognised and treated.

Good Mother myths and misogyny work hand in hand to make birth a dreadful, damaging – even deadly – experience for many women. Abuse and neglect can be justified and ignored where women, particularly marginalised women, are regarded with contempt. Good Mother myths of self-sacrifice mean that women can be railroaded and ignored. Women are givers who must subordinate their bodies not just to their children but also their healthcare providers. And then there is the culture of mother blame to throw into the mix, where women are blamed and blame themselves for difficult birth experiences.

Birth, like everything else we've considered in this book, needs to be viewed on a broader canvas. Making birth better has to be part of remaking motherhood. This is the hope which mother-dom can inspire.

4

Feeding Frenzy

'Breast milk is every baby's birthright. Nature has provided this food for his protection, and the mother who denies it to him without good reason is *stealing* [original emphasis] from her baby.' This was the claim of a manual on natural childbirth first published in 1948.[1]

Judgements about breastfeeding are grounded in deep-seated beliefs about women as givers. Indeed, a 2018 UNICEF report is called *Breastfeeding: A Mother's Gift, for Every Child*. This unfairly suggests that breastfeeding is always within a mother's gift (which it is not, for many reasons which we shall come on to). It also implies that mothers who do not breastfeed are selfishly withholding something precious from their child.[2]

But breastfeeding is not the only thing women are expected to give. There are competing claims on women's bodies – breasts are for babies, breasts are for men. Women can never win. A qualitative study among women in North West England found that however women fed their baby, they were made to feel selfish: women who formula-fed for depriving their baby of their breast milk, mothers who breastfed because others, such as partners and grandparents, were not able to feed the baby. Both breast-feeding and formula-feeding mothers recounted feelings of humiliation, fear, inferiority and inadequacy.[3]

It is acceptable to censure and shame mothers about any aspect of child-rearing, but feeding is a particularly charged issue.

Breastfeeding carries a tangled mess of contradictions. Women have to navigate powerful visions of breastfeeding as natural, but also bottle-feeding as the norm. The campaigner and author Gabrielle Palmer highlights that images of bottle-feeding are all around us, including the universal bottle signs outside baby care rooms in shops and airports.[4]

Breastfeeding signifies the power of women's bodies to sustain their babies, taking control away from medical professionals, men and formula companies. Jennifer Nash highlights the radical potential of breastfeeding as 'Black maternal commitment to Black life'. Black mothers are positioned at 'the front line of securing Black life, with Black breasts becoming a key technology – the key technology – to immunize Black children from physical and psychic violence'.[5]

But breastfeeding also bolsters beliefs that it is women's natural role to look after babies and requires women to relinquish their bodily autonomy. It fuels the Good Mother myths of unconditional sacrifice and joyful giving. Ambivalent or negative feelings, as we shall see, are often not acknowledged or sanctioned.

A Delightful Duty

Similar to other aspects of mothering, women have to contend with Good Mother myths which not only prescribe how they should feed but also how they should feel. In her review of nineteenth-century advice written by mothers and doctors, Berit Åström was only able to find one work with a negative view of breastfeeding – *Mrs Beeton's Book of Household Management*. Mrs Beeton described breastfeeding as 'privation and penance' and recommended introducing supplementary food at an early age so the mother has the 'liberty to go out for business or pleasure'.

This went against the grain of other advice books, where, Åström notes, it was 'taken as self-evident that breastfeeding is an emotionally fulfilling activity'. Thomas Graham, a Scottish physician, described it as a 'delightful duty' and claimed that 'no earthly pleasure of the fond mother can equal'. As Åström points out, this echoes the tone of modern-day advocates of breastfeeding, such as La Leche League, who we shall come to shortly.[6]

Despite breastfeeding being presented as a 'delightful duty', it was thought necessary to instruct women to keep their emotions in check when feeding. The popular Victorian work we encountered in Chapter 1, *The Management of Infancy: Physiological and Moral*, warned against 'vivid mental emotion' in nursing mothers. It advocated 'habitual equanimity of temper' and recounted the cautionary tale of the carpenter's wife who tried to break up a fight between her husband and a soldier who was brandishing a sword at him. She took the sword from the soldier and, the reader is informed, broke it into pieces. Straight afterwards, the carpenter's wife put her baby to her breast 'and by so doing sealed its fate. In a few minutes, the infant left off sucking, became restless, panted, and *sank dead on its mother's bosom* [italics in the original].' The book employs the classic expert tactic of trying to control women with the threat of dire consequences for their babies. The authors caution:

> Perpetually recurring fits of bad temper . . . produce similar affects in a more slow and gradual manner, but with almost equal certainty – and if anything can exert a salutary influence on mothers who are prone to the indulgence of passion, it must be the contemplation of such a case as that of the carpenter's wife.[7]

Directives about breastfeeding have changed over time. As we saw in Chapter 1, in the first half of the twentieth century women were urged to feed their babies according to strict schedules to ensure good character. Eric Pritchard, the doctor and author of infant care books we met in the first chapter, was a strong proponent of scheduled feeds. He gave this impressive sounding but nonsensical scientific justification for keeping feeds regular:

There is a reasonable probability that the receptive and impressionable nerve centres which control the functions of mammary secretion will acquire a rhythm and automatism which can be made to subserve most useful purposes, and promote the chances of successful breast-feeding.

This is, of course, contrary to everything we know about the physiology of breastfeeding (frequent feeding stimulates milk supply). As well as cloaking his arguments in dubious science, Pritchard issued the customary grim warnings – women feeding their babies too much or too frequently caused them to 'die in shoals'. Pritchard also echoed earlier experts on the importance of emotional restraint. He claimed that a woman's psychological influence is critical to successfully feeding infants and had particular faith in what he called 'the complacent and so-called cow-like woman'.[8]

While feeding advice is now grounded in the physiology of breastfeeding, it is still strongly prescriptive and is applied to bottle-feeding as well. A guide for health professionals on infant feeding, published by the charity First Steps Nutrition Trust, stresses the importance of 'responsive' feeding. On the face of it, this sounds sensible – recognising when babies need to be fed and when they are full. But the word 'responsive' has been stretched to cover how women interact with their babies. There is a list of things women should do 'to encourage responsiveness and discourage overfeeding'. The very first instruction is 'hold the baby close and look into their eyes during feeds'. This comes before recognising the signs that the baby is hungry or full.[9]

The dictate to look into a baby's eyes during feeding can lead to confusion and guilt. I have had women asking me if it is normal that their baby doesn't look at them when they feed them. In a US study on breastfeeding among autistic women, one mother reported concentrating on her phone to cope with feelings of overstimulation, commenting, 'But I know some people look down on this because it limits eye contact.'[10]

There is nothing innate, instinctual or inevitable about mothers and babies gazing into each other's eyes during feeding. This is a Good Mother myth. As the anthropologist David Lancy says, 'The ethnographic record is quite consistent in showing mothers frequently nursing infants but, otherwise, paying them relatively little attention.'[11] Indeed, in Nso society in the northwest of Cameroon, mothers positively discourage their babies from looking at them during breastfeeding by blowing air into their eyes. This is to school babies in cultural norms about avoiding direct eye contact.[12] Breastfeeding is portrayed as universal but, like all aspects of motherhood, it is strongly shaped by context, circumstances and culture.

The Most Natural Thing in the World?

Breastfeeding advocates can frame practices driven by deeply pragmatic considerations as timeless and natural. But forager societies do not choose around-the-clock feeding and extended breastfeeding because they are vessels of eternal truth about human nature. Highly dependent babies and young children are a burden for people constantly on the move in pursuit of food, so long intervals between births are better. Continual and extended breastfeeding, along with taboos against sex after childbirth, are strategies to control fertility.[13]

There are wide variations over time and across cultures in how babies are fed. For instance, the anthropologist Kirsten Hastrup documents the long period of history in Iceland – from sometime in the sixteenth century to well into the nineteenth century – when women did not breastfeed their babies beyond the first few days of life. Instead, babies were given cow's milk or, if the family could afford it, cream, both of which were seen to be better than breast milk. At a time of widespread impoverishment in Icelandic society, cream was particularly valued as a symbol of wealth and success. Mortality rates were, unsurprisingly, very high.[14]

The way in which breastfeeding is portrayed as 'natural' is a culturally specific Good Mother myth. In her history of breast-feeding in America, the historian Jessica Martucci argues that in the West breastfeeding has been 'explicitly marked as "natural" since male scholars in the age of the scientific revolution began carving the world into separate poles of machine/male and nature/female'. But, as Martucci points out, 'what exactly it has meant to call something "natural" . . . has varied'. Martucci explains how breastfeeding was central to an ideology of natural motherhood which was regarded as a bulwark against the erosion of traditional gender roles in the post–Second World War era. Breastfeeding was portrayed as 'a universal salve for a host of modern "problems", a list that could encompass anything from homosexuality to divorce'.[15] As we shall go on to see, magical thinking about the capacity of breastfeeding to tackle society's ills continues to endure.

La Leche League, an organisation founded in America in 1956 to provide woman-to-woman support for breastfeeding, has been one of the strongest exponents of the naturalness of breast-feeding. *The Womanly Art of Breastfeeding*, first published in 1958, repeatedly invokes 'Nature'. The most recent edition states: 'Nature has given both you and your baby the instincts and skills that can help you overcome any early challenges you might face.' Formula-feeding is characterised as 'fooling nature' and separating mothers and babies at night is 'not at all what Nature had in mind'.[16] As this demonstrates, equating breastfeeding with 'nature' can be used to justify a series of generalisations and directives.

The history of La Leche League illustrates how narratives about 'nature' are in fact deeply grounded in a particular world-view. The League was founded by a group of Catholic mothers, and its name comes from a shrine to the Madonna in Florida, called Nuestra Señora de La Leche y Buen Parto (which the League loosely translates as meaning 'Our Lady of Happy Delivery and Plentiful Milk'). In her history of the movement, the writer Jule DeJager Ward argues that the League's philosophy is infused with a distinctively American Catholic outlook; biology is the foundation of moral obligation, love is service to others and evangelisation is practised through example.

Central to La Leche League's philosophy, Ward observes, is the belief that 'were it not for an intrusive culture, a woman's natural instincts would enable her to make morally correct choices about infant and childcare'. She comments that the League is lacking 'the critical self-awareness' to give personal, economic and cultural factors due consideration.[17] This attitude is neatly illustrated when *The Womanly Art of Breastfeeding* blithely claims: 'Even with a challenging situation, breastfeeding often makes life easier.'

The association of breastfeeding with nature and the primitive can be particularly problematic for Black women, evoking stereotypes of animal-like sexuality, which have deep roots in the scientific racism used to justify slavery and racial oppression. Legal scholar Andrea Freeman highlights the link between Black women's low breastfeeding rates and slavery. She notes that 'the most common image of a Black woman nursing, then [that is, in the twentieth century] and now, is not of a nurturing, middle-class African American but, instead, of a bare-breasted African woman. These types of images . . . make breastfeeding by Black women appear to be a primitive practice.'[18] These associations have been challenged by Black women. Jennifer Nash explains how, in the photography of the artist and activist Lakisha Cohill, a 'fictionalised Africa, an imagined natural past, becomes a source of strength and empowerment'.[19]

'A common shared experience in the Black culture . . . is kept alive in the oral histories and attitudes of African American women' concluded the midwife and academic Stephanie DeVane-Johnson in her research among African American women aged eighteen to fifty-one in North Carolina. The association of breastfeeding with slavery and forced wet nursing had discouraged older women from breastfeeding, while younger women were put off breastfeeding because it is seen as 'nasty'. Some saw formula-feeding as a more empowering option. One woman said: 'I have a choice today. I don't have to work in someone's house and clean. I don't have to breastfeed if I don't want to, so I choose not to breastfeed.'[20]

The sociologist Linda Blum found similar themes in her qualitative research in the 1990s with working-class African American women. Most of the women in her study did not breastfeed, regarding bottle-feeding as a better option because of factors such as stressful lives and health problems. Some also explicitly rejected the 'animal-like' aspects of breastfeeding, while others hinted at it. One woman quipped, 'The *natural* thing to me was to bottlefeed.'[21]

The association of breastfeeding with animals has stirred up ambivalent and negative feelings throughout history. In Greek and Latin literature, the classicist Patricia Salzman-Mitchell observes that male authors 'express discomfort regarding a practice that seems unknown, even taboo, with a hue of incest, close to the animal side of nature, rather than to the civilized world, and present women as mysterious, polluting, dangerous and different'.

Despite this discomfort, women were urged to breastfeed. The philosophical and moral texts of Rome, such as those of Plutarch, Tacitus and Aulus Gellius, argued that breastfeeding forges strong bonds between mother and child and strengthens the character of the infant. However, it seems that Roman women, or at least those who could afford to, ignored these dictates. For instance, Soranus, the author of several medical treatises, sets out extensive recommendations on selecting a wet nurse, illustrating that commercial wet nursing was common in Rome among the upper classes.[22]

As we saw in Chapter 1, wet nursing was also the norm in France for centuries. Élisabeth Badinter relates how breastfeeding was believed to be physically bad for mothers in seventeenth- and eighteenth-century France. It was regarded as inappropriate for noble women because of its association with animals and was considered immodest. She observes that in letters and memoirs, the word 'ridiculous' was frequently used to describe breastfeeding.[23]

However, as we have explored in Chapter 1, what is 'natural' is now unthinkingly and automatically deemed to be desirable. The portrayal of breastfeeding as natural carries the connotation that women who don't breastfeed are, in some sense, unnatural. This can fuel the moral outrage which women can be subjected to either explicitly or more obliquely. It can also lead to women judging themselves harshly. The writer Emma Jane Unsworth observes, 'There is propaganda everywhere featuring the word "natural", and a resulting sense of failure for those who don't breastfeed.'[24]

Breastfeeding Realities

Assumptions that breastfeeding is a natural part of motherhood, and a woman's gift to give, are profoundly unfair. There are many reasons why women do not want to or cannot breastfeed. Women's economic and social circumstances can make breast-feeding impractical or even impossible. As Linda Blum's research has found, formula-feeding is more feasible for women with busy and stressful lives. In the West, breastfeeding rates are greater among higher-income women, who have more resources to pay for breastfeeding support and can afford longer periods of maternity leave.[25] In her qualitative study of first-time, middle-class mothers in San Francisco, the sociologist Orit Avishai found they spent hundreds of dollars on items such as nursing bras, breast pumps, nursing pillows and chairs.[26]

Barriers to breastfeeding are not just economic. For some women, the thought of breastfeeding is unbearable because of experiences of abuse, violence or birth trauma. In one study, a woman who had been sexually abused as a child disclosed, 'When I placed my baby to the breast, it triggered flashbacks of my abuse as a child.'[27]

Women with disabilities or chronic health conditions can find that pain, fatigue and difficulties holding their baby to feed can make breastfeeding challenging, if not impossible. One woman living with quadriplegia participating in a Canadian study said, 'I didn't realize how hard it would be to hold my son. I thought I can put my arms together and that would kind of work . . . You have to really support their head and I didn't have the ability to do that.'[28]

Feelings of guilt and shame can lead to women running risks to their health. A mother with autoimmune rheumatic disease who had twins recounted how 'I was in a lot of pain and I was struggling to hold two babies to breastfeed as well because my joints were sore . . . I marched on and then at six weeks I dropped a child.' She found life became easier when she stopped breastfeeding:

> I was so desperate to do what I'd thought was right with these two tiny little babies, but actually as soon as I did give up breastfeeding . . . suddenly being a mum was so much more fun and I had two much happier babies because I was much more settled.[29]

As this illustrates, the Good Mother myth that breastfeeding is natural and enjoyable is highly problematic. For some women, breastfeeding is rewarding and pleasurable. But universal claims ignore and erase the rich complexity of women's experiences. Feelings about breastfeeding can be negative or ambivalent. A woman may find breastfeeding delightful one day and suffocating the next.

Although breastfeeding is promoted as being good for bonding with the baby, for some women it can be the absolute opposite. Emma Jane Unsworth writes, 'Breastfeeding didn't bond me to my baby. It made me hate my baby.'[30] In a qualitative study of Icelandic mothers, one woman recalled:

> This was a really bad period for me, the baby and my partner. During this time I was kind of just 'plugging away' with the breastfeeding. Every hour in the day revolved around trying to

feed my son. I didn't really know this child, I was just either waking him up, trying to get him to sleep, pumping or feeding him from the breast or the bottle. There was no time to look at the baby, enjoy holding him and being his mother.[31]

There is little acknowledgement of the emotional complexities of breastfeeding in breastfeeding advocacy or literature. The changing advice of Dr Spock provides a good example of how the cultural acceptability of negative emotions has lessened. The researcher Stephanie Knaak observes that in the 1946 edition of *The Common Sense Book of Baby and Child Care*, Dr Spock advised that women who feel a sense of revulsion about breastfeeding should bottle-feed, otherwise 'it may disturb the mother's relationship to her child, and do more harm than good.' In the 1998 edition, Spock says mothers should use their own judgement, but encourages them to press on with breastfeeding by stating 'it is too seldom mentioned that, after a couple of weeks, breast-feeding becomes definitely pleasurable for the mother.'[32]

Framing breastfeeding as natural doesn't just foreclose the possibility of negative feelings. Being natural is also associated with being effortless; we describe something as 'coming naturally' to someone if it seems easy to them. With breastfeeding, this can lead to the assumption that it should be straightforward and that women do not need help or support. As the public health researcher Amy Brown says, feeding difficulties are often glossed over so women are not put off breastfeeding:

We effectively shield mothers from the idea of potential difficulties, demands or inconveniences to encourage them to breastfeed, but it has the opposite effect, leaving them shocked and concerned that because these issues haven't been mentioned, something must be wrong.

There are many factors which can make breastfeeding difficult. A lack of knowledge about typical baby feeding patterns (frequent and changeable) can undermine women's confidence. This is particularly the case if people around them make unhelpful comments like, 'Why is that baby hungry again so soon?'[33] Women can feel under pressure to put their baby into a routine or to try to get the baby to sleep better at night. There are taboos about breasts being on show and a sense that women should be trying to 'get their bodies back' after pregnancy. As Brown points out, these societal expectations can discourage women from feeding their babies when they need to be fed, which can inhibit milk supply and lead to problems such as mastitis (inflammation of the breast tissue).

This all takes place against a backdrop of formula promotion and cultural perceptions of formula as the norm. In a BBC *Woman's Hour* survey of 1,162 UK women who had had a baby in the last ten years, 19% of mothers who formula-fed had felt pressure from family or friends to feed their baby formula.[34]

Many women stop breastfeeding before they want to (which should *not* be confused with thinking that all women want to breastfeed). Large-scale surveys run in the US and the UK found that around three-fifths of women did not breastfeed for as long as they would have liked.[35] In the UK survey, the figure rose to 86% of women who breastfed for between one and two weeks.[36]

It can be difficult to get the help and support which can be needed for breastfeeding to go smoothly. Three-quarters (74%) of respondents in a survey of Mumsnet users agreed, 'There's too much emphasis on telling women why they should breastfeed, and not enough on supporting them to breastfeed.' Among women who tried to establish breastfeeding in the first twenty-four hours after birth, 29% rated healthcare support as poor or terrible.[37] In an international online study among 679 mothers of babies under six months who had initiated breastfeeding, only 57% felt well supported by health professionals on infant feeding issues. The remainder (43%) reported feeling moderately to not at all supported.[38] Birthrights' inquiry into racial injustice in maternity care found that assumptions that Black or Brown women would know how to breastfeed or would have a lot of family support made it harder for them to access help. One woman was told 'you African women know what you are doing'.[39]

Conflicting advice is a common problem; for instance, whether or not to offer both breasts, how long a baby should feed, waking a sleeping baby or leaving them be, avoiding or embracing nipple shields. A common complaint in my postnatal groups is being told different things by different people. In an NCT study about postnatal care, one woman said, 'Every single health worker or midwife I spoke to both in hospital and afterwards at home had different advice to give.' Another woman was advised to have skin-to-skin contact with her baby after the birth and wait for the baby to find the nipple: 'Two minutes later another midwife came in and asked me what I was doing and why I wasn't guiding my baby to the nipple when she was obviously hungry.'[40]

As this illustrates, advice can be imperious and unhelpful. When breastfeeding my newborn baby in hospital, I was told by a health professional that I was 'doing it wrong', but I wasn't told why or what I should be doing instead. The experience was bewildering and upsetting. I have heard distressing stories from women who have felt belittled and demoralised by health professionals. A woman in one of my postnatal groups was told to put her baby to her breast after the baby was vaccinated even though, to her anguish, she had not been able to breastfeed.

Another disturbing experience for women is being touched without consent. In the North West England feeding study referred to earlier in this chapter, women described how they had had their breasts handled by health professionals which for some 'induced intense distress and humiliation'. One woman recounted how a midwife got hold of her breast and squeezed it to demonstrate how breastfeeding works. Another woman described how a midwife, without explanation, pulled her gown down, rubbed the baby's head 'dead hard into my boob' until she latched on and then walked off.[41] For women bearing the scars of abuse or trauma, or who have sensory issues about being touched, these sorts of experiences can be particularly distressing.

The Myth of Enough Milk

As part of the general practice of glossing over potential difficulties, women are routinely told that breastfeeding is possible for most women.[42] For instance, the NHS website says that 'nearly all women produce enough milk for their baby'.[43] In reality, not producing enough milk is why many women stop breastfeeding. Indeed, this was the most common reason given in national feeding surveys conducted in Australia and the UK.[44] In the US survey referred to earlier, 58% of women who did not breastfeed for as long as they would have liked said they stopped because they did not have enough milk.[45]

There are plenty of social and physiological factors that can inhibit a woman's milk supply, such as too long between feeds and topping up with formula. If the baby is not transferring milk properly (for example, because of tongue tie, illness or pain), this can impact milk supply. For women with physical disabilities, delays in finding the right adaptations or equipment to breastfeed can lead to their milk supply drying up.[46]

I also suspect that another issue is that cultural pressures to breastfeed mean that it is more acceptable for women to say they are not breastfeeding because they didn't have enough milk instead of having to disclose that they didn't actually want to. It can be an effective way to duck Good Mother myths about breastfeeding.

But there are some women who still do not produce enough milk for their babies even if none of these factors exist. In one of those delightful medical terms that seems designed to make women feel bad about themselves, this is known as 'primary lactation failure'.

There are a number of reasons why breastfeeding may not be physically possible. These include hormonal complications, which may be linked to polycystic ovarian syndrome, thyroid abnormalities, diabetes or gestational diabetes and insufficient glandular tissue developing during adolescence (also known as mammary hypoplasia).[47]

Because of the hegemony of breastfeeding ideology, this information is usually hidden away. The paediatrician Marianne Neifert contrasts the portrayal of breastfeeding with other bodily activities:

> The bold claims made about the infallibility of lactation are not cited about any other physiologic processes. A health care professional would never tell a diabetic woman that 'every pancreas can make insulin' or insist to a devastated infertility patient that 'every woman can get pregnant'. The fact is that lactation, like all physiologic functions, sometimes fails because of various medical causes.[48]

We don't know how many women are affected by these issues because the research hasn't been done. The Infant Feeding Practices Study, a longitudinal study of US women, found that 12% of the 2,335 women surveyed experienced what the researchers called 'disrupted lactation', (it's a better phrase than 'primary lactation failure') where women stopped breastfeeding before they wanted to because of difficulties with latch, pain and milk supply. Given how many barriers to breastfeeding there are, the authors acknowledge that it is hard to estimate the 'real' prevalence of disrupted lactation.[49] Amy Brown estimates that between 1 and 2% of women are physiologically unable to breastfeed, noting that this fits with the figure of 98% initiation in countries where breastfeeding is the norm. However, she concedes that the origins of this figure are 'slightly mysterious'.[50]

Even if it is only 1% of women who are physiologically unable to breastfeed, that it still an awful lot of women who may be left devastated if they can't breastfeed and believe that this is their fault. The sense that breastfeeding is generally possible if you just try hard enough is implied in some breastfeeding advocacy. *The Womanly Art of Breastfeeding* urges women experiencing breastfeeding difficulties not to give up: 'Most women who "can't" breastfeed simply don't have enough information or support . . .

If your helper is out of ideas and things still aren't working, ask her to refer you to another resource. There's almost always something more that can be done.'

Women can go to astonishing lengths to try to get breastfeeding to work. In the 'disrupted lactation' study the researchers said:

> In our clinical work with breastfeeding mothers, we regularly encounter women who have taken extraordinary measures to breastfeed. Women visit multiple specialists, ingest countless herbal preparations, and endure every-hour pumping regimens, supplemental nursing systems, and topical ointments in an effort to establish a normal breastfeeding relationship.[51]

It is profoundly unfair to women not to be honest that breastfeeding may not be possible. For instance, there is nothing on the NHS's website that mentions that there may be physiological issues which lead to insufficient milk supply.[52] In cases of what the UK's National Institute for Health and Care Excellence calls 'maternal prolactin deficiency', the recommended approach is referral to an endocrinologist.[53] But this information is in a clinical knowledge summary – so is targeted at health professionals, not the public.

Women are, in effect, told to just get on with it. Elaine Kasket, a writer and psychologist, recounts being ordered by a health visitor to hide the formula away 'so you won't be tempted' and advised to cut two holes in a T-shirt: 'Just let them hang out so you're always ready. No formula, no bottles. Everything will be fine – as long as you persist.' The next health visitor to visit was horrified: 'You need to take your baby to the hospital immediately,' she said. 'Take her now. Your daughter is starving to death.'[54]

It is this sort of experience that has sparked the 'fed is best' movement. The Fed Is Best Foundation was set up by Christie del Castillo-Hegyi, whose son suffered newborn jaundice, hypoglycaemia and severe dehydration due to insufficient milk intake from exclusive breastfeeding. He is now neurologically disabled.[55] Of course, the argument that 'fed is best' can also be used to pressurise women. Women are told to give up breastfeeding, rather than offered practical and emotional support to continue.

We need to know more about why some women find breast-feeding such a struggle, whatever they do or try. In *Invisible Women: Exposing Data Bias in a World Designed for Men*, writer and campaigner Caroline Criado Perez highlights the absence of research into medical issues that mainly or only affect women. For example, premenstrual syndrome, which can be a debilitating condition, is 'chronically under-studied', with one 2016 analysis finding that there are five times as many studies on erectile dysfunction as premenstrual syndrome.[56]

Breastfeeding is also woefully under-researched. A review of herbal and pharmaceutical remedies to increase milk pro-duction found a lack of high-quality research and insufficient information to guide clinical recommendations.[57] A Cochrane Review into the impact of extra fluids on milk production found just one small research trial of 210 women which had been done in the 1950s and was judged to be of low quality.[58] Another Cochrane Review found a lack of robust research on what can help with engorgement, where breasts feel uncomfortably hard and full of milk.[59]

We need much more research into breastfeeding. As Amy Brown rightly asks:

> Given the breadth and depth of medical knowledge, why do women still not have answers if they can't breastfeed? . . . As with any other bodily function, the breast deserves a bank of research and knowledge to enable it to function well, and answers and treatment options if it does not.[60]

The Science of Breastfeeding

Nature is one pillar in prescribing how women should feed their babies. Science provides the other. The scientific consensus around breastfeeding can leave women feeling that they are harming their babies for life if they are not breastfed. As I heard one woman put it, half-jokingly, 'I've given my baby formula, he's going to die early and be fat and stupid.'

But is the evidence as strong as we are led to believe? The academic Joan Wolf has described the science behind the consensus in favour of breastfeeding as 'deeply problematic' and the benefits 'marginal' for most babies in the developed world. Her review of breastfeeding research concludes that while there is compelling evidence that it reduces gastrointestinal infections, the evidence for other benefits is contradictory: 'For every piece of research linking it to better health, another finds it to be irrelevant, weakly significant, or inextricably tied to factors that are difficult to measure with the standard tools of science.' She argues that research simply cannot eliminate the possibility that breastfeeding is an indicator of parents' general commitment to healthy living, rather than having a positive impact in and of itself.[61]

Emily Oster, an economist, comes to similar conclusions: 'It seems reasonable to conclude that breastfeeding lowers infant eczema and gastrointestinal infections. For the other illness outcomes, the most compelling evidence is in favour of a small reduction in ear infections in breastfed children.' In terms of long-term benefits, 'the data does not provide strong evidence for long-term health or cognitive benefits of breastfeeding for your child'. On sudden infant death syndrome (SIDS), Oster explores case-control studies (where babies who have died from SIDS are compared with babies who have not) which show that babies who have died are less likely to have been breastfed. Oster argues that there are important differences between the two groups of babies that have nothing to do with breastfeeding. When studies take into account risk factors such as smoking or prematurity, the effects are much smaller or disappear altogether.[62]

Against this, a 2016 *Lancet* paper which examined twenty-eight systematic reviews and meta-analyses found a range of benefits for breastfeeding in both developed and developing countries. These were protection against diarrhoea, respiratory infections, ear infections, malocclusion (where the teeth are not aligned properly), increased intelligence and probable reductions in obesity and diabetes. There was no link found between breast-feeding and food allergies, asthma or eczema (note that Oster thought there was evidence of this) or with blood pressure or cholesterol.[63] Although the reductions in obesity and diabetes were only judged to be 'probable', there is no such ambivalence in much breastfeeding promotion. The World Health Organiza-tion's website states: 'Breastfed children perform better on intelligence tests, are less likely to be overweight or obese and less prone to diabetes later in life.'[64]

No wonder women equate formula-feeding with producing stupid and unhealthy children. However, the differences in IQ are modest and are not found in all studies. In the sixteen studies included in the *Lancet* paper, children who were breastfed had IQs which were higher on average by 3.4 points. Only nine of the studies adjusted for maternal intelligence, which is known to be associated with children's IQ, and these showed a smaller difference of 2.6 points. Two to three points is not going to make much differ-ence to how an individual child's IQ is classified. The average IQ sits within a range of 90–109 and other bands span ten points (high average is 110–19). Emily Oster points to studies comparing chil-dren who were breastfed to siblings who were not which have found no relationship between breastfeeding and IQ.[65] This supports the argument that it is something about the family environment more generally that is driving the relationship between breastfeeding and IQ. Or it may be, as Amy Brown argues in relation to one sibling study, that the research is flawed because it does not consider exclu-sive breastfeeding or take into account duration of breastfeeding.[66]

At a public health level, the promotion of breastfeeding makes sense. Even a small benefit can be valuable when it is multiplied across a population, and breast milk contains biologically active compounds which may have benefits that we do not yet understand and cannot measure. The authors of the *Lancet* paper suggest that 'crucial imprinting events might be modulated during breastfeeding, with potential lifelong effects for the infant' through the impact of a mother's individually tailored breast milk on an infant's gut.

But we are still a long way off being able to show that, as is speculated in the *Lancet* paper, breast milk is 'probably the most specific personalised medicine' that a child is likely to receive.[67] Incidentally, some studies on the properties of breast milk have been conducted among primates and rats. As with other elements of child-rearing, we need to watch out for animal studies being used to pontificate about humans.

The research needs to continue, while taking steps to disentangle issues such as the duration of breastfeeding. However, we also need to be careful not to let magical thinking about breastfeeding's impact on children's happiness and health distort our investigations of the benefits of breast milk.

A Better Formula for Information

One of the issues with the evidence base is that we don't know – but categorically should – the impact of formula milk not being made up properly. The UK's All-Party Parliamentary Group on Infant Feeding and Inequalities has concluded that research is 'urgently needed' into the extent of unsafe formula use among low-income and vulnerable families and the risks this poses to health. The report shared anecdotal evidence of low-income families having to resort to risky practices such as watering down feeds to make supplies of formula last longer, not throwing away unused formula after a feed, adding cereal to bottles to bulk up the feed or giving young babies cow's milk.[68]

We don't know how many babies are getting sick because formula is too expensive or information on how to use formula safely is withheld to even out the playing field given the marketing might of formula companies. We have every reason not to trust them. The central insight of Gabrielle Palmer's *The Politics of Breastfeeding*, which has inspired generations of activists, is that companies that sell formula milk and bottles 'benefit financially from keeping breastfeeding in check'.[69]

Formula milk was aggressively marketed in the developing world in the 1970s. Tactics such as dressing saleswomen in nurses' uniforms encouraged mothers to choose bottle-feeding. Because of poor sanitation and impure water, this led to malnutrition, diarrhoea and death. Following a high-profile boycott between 1977 and 1984, Nestlé agreed to follow the World Health Organization's International Code of Marketing of Breastmilk Substitutes. This code prohibits the advertising of formula in public services, providing free samples of formula to health professionals or mothers and giving out promotional items.[70]

The pushback against formula companies has fundamentally changed perceptions of formula milk. Today it is hard to imagine a book on breastfeeding including a chapter entitled 'Is Human Milk Good Enough for Babies?' as Sheila Kitzinger's *The Experience of Breastfeeding* did in 1987.[71]

But formula companies still benefit from keeping breastfeeding at bay. There is evidence that they continue to provide gifts, samples and promotional materials to health professionals.[72] And breastfeeding can be subtly undermined in their advertising campaigns. For instance, one TV advert which ran in the UK, US and Australia shows a breastfeeding woman in a shirt with buttons, a highly impractical item of clothing for breastfeeding. The top part of the shirt is awkwardly pushed down, exposing her shoulder. It imperceptibly associates breastfeeding with nudity and evokes taboos against breasts being visible.

The Baby Friendly Initiative, a global programme of the World Health Organization and UNICEF, was introduced in 1992 to keep formula companies out of maternity services. But the Baby Friendly standards can problematise formula-feeding to the detriment of mothers. There can be something of a Voldemort approach taken, where formula milk is the thing-that-shall-not-be-named. The Baby Friendly guidance does say that mothers should be given 'adequate information on how to make up a feed, preferably 1-2-1, in the early postnatal period'. However, it is deemed unacceptable to provide information on bottle-feeding in a group setting antenatally or postnatally to groups which include mothers who are breastfeeding. To do so, it is argued, will result in 'reinforcing bottle-feeding as the cultural norm and giving the impression that all mothers need this information'.[73]

These sorts of directives are stigmatising and shaming. The North West England feeding study found that restrictions on being able to discuss formula-feeding left women feeling 'dejected and isolated'.[74] In a Scottish study entitled *The Midwives Aren't Allowed to Tell You*, midwives were seen to be reluctant to give advice about formula-feeding. There was a lack of information on how to prepare bottle-feeds and how much to feed the baby. Pressure was sometimes strongly applied. One woman said: 'I wanted to give up in the hospital . . . I couldn't get any sleep, I had a C-section and my third night there I was like, "I want to change to bottle", and the midwife told me I wasn't allowed.'[75]

Women deserve unbiased and non-judgemental information on feeding and safe formula preparation. The Voldemort approach to formula-feeding – treating it as the appalling thing-that-should-not-be-named – infantilises women and is disrespectful. It is reflective of how the whole issue of infant feeding is approached – playing down difficulties and discouraging alternatives in an attempt to push women down a breastfeeding path.

Similar dynamics are at play when we consider what information is available for women who want to stop breastfeeding. As well as undercutting women's wishes, a lack of information could also potentially put their health at risk because suddenly stopping can lead to blocked ducts and mastitis. There are many reasons why women may need to stop breastfeeding quickly – going back to work, starting on medication, a hospital stay, a trip away from their baby. But the way this whole topic is treated illustrates how information about breastfeeding is shrouded in pressure and moralising. Until 2017, there was no information at all on the NHS website about stopping breastfeeding. Now there is, but first you have to scroll through recommendations to breastfeed.[76] Other websites present the information along the lines of 'are you sure you really want to stop?' This may be helpful for a mother who is having doubts about her decision or is being pressured but does nothing for women who have come to the end of the road with breastfeeding.[77]

La Leche League's information, in particular, is spectacularly unhelpful. It warns against ending breastfeeding 'abruptly' and claims: 'Since it is normal for babies to continue to breastfeed into the second year or beyond, the weaning period may last months or years.'[78] The League recommends 'natural weaning', appearing to be unaware of 'weaning conflict', where the mother and child have different perspectives on the timing of weaning.[79] Children being forcibly weaned is a well-known phenomenon in many cultures. For instance, a 1960s study documented how toddlers from Tarong in the Philippines were discouraged from nursing by the spectre of the Wawak, a spirit who kills and eats bad children. Mothers also put pepper or manure on their breasts to discourage feeding.[80]

Feeding Judgements

'There's so much pressure on you to breastfeed,' observed a woman taking part in a UK qualitative study. She went on to say, 'You're told that breast is best and you should do it and so when you don't you think you are a failure and it's what you should be doing.'[81]

Women in the North West England feeding study recounted how health professionals made them feel 'second best', like a 'bad mother' who was 'denying' and 'depriving' their child because they were not breastfeeding.[82] An international online survey among 601 mothers of babies under six months who were formula-feeding found that two-thirds said they had experienced feelings of guilt (67%) and stigma (68%), and three-quarters (76%) felt the need to defend their decision to use formula. Women who wished to breastfeed during pregnancy or had initiated it were more susceptible to guilt, whereas those who had planned to formula-feed or were exclusively formula-feeding from birth were more likely to feel stigma.[83]

Although women are put under a huge amount of pressure to breastfeed, there is a very narrow scope of what is deemed acceptable. This is another double bind to contend with. Women breastfeeding in public can be a particular trigger for judgement, disapproval and misogyny, revealing deep-rooted views about what women's breasts are for. Public health researcher Aimee Grant analysed the comments posted in response to a *Daily Mail* article about a protest supporting women's right to breastfeed in public. Women who breastfed in public were variously described as exhibitionist, unattractive, lazy, bad parents and lacking in self-respect. The belief that breastfeeding in public is exhibitionist is bizarre. I suspect that people who think this are projecting their own feelings about breasts onto the woman feeding her child.

Even stranger are the comments describing the protesters as 'flashers' and claiming they were inviting sexual contact from men.[84] Sheila Kitzinger argued that feelings of disgust about breastfeeding are closely connected to the view of a woman's body as male property: 'It turns out that men are the ultimate arbiters about what we do with our breasts.'[85]

Where breastfeeding in public happens makes a difference to some people's views. A YouGov survey of 1,869 British adults found that while most thought it is generally acceptable for women to breastfeed their child in public (77% agreed, but 18% thought it unacceptable), levels of tolerance varied according to location. The beach (84%) or a park bench (79%) are, it transpires, much more acceptable than a restaurant (59%).[86] There is no logic at all to thinking that feeding a baby in a place where everyone else is eating is less acceptable. It is illustrative of our peculiar attitudes towards breastfeeding.

Some people would rather women who breastfeed their babies remove themselves from public spaces altogether. For instance, a grandmother taking part in an Australian study said, 'The politician that wanted to feed her baby in parliament and things like that, I don't think she needed to make that statement, there was no need for it, she didn't need to take the baby in and feed it.' It is apparently hard for some people to comprehend that a woman is simply feeding her baby while getting on with her daily life. Instead, this is implausibly construed as some sort of public performance.[87]

These sorts of beliefs constrain women. In the BBC *Woman's Hour* survey referred to earlier, 30% of mothers who formula-fed said they would have liked to have breastfed their baby but felt embarrassed about doing so in public. Women who do breastfeed can be isolated in their homes, particularly in the early days, when latching the baby onto the breast can be tricky and several attempts are needed.

Judgement and disapproval also come in spades when women breastfeed children beyond the first few months of babyhood. In the North West England study, women breastfeeding toddlers felt castigated as 'hippies', 'weirdoes' or 'naturalists'.[88] In another English study, one woman recounted getting dirty looks and said, 'The only media coverage they show of breast-feeders are women still breastfeeding their eight-year-old children that are really extreme stories designed to make breast-feeders look like sort of weird freaky paedophiles.'[89]

Although I have been very critical of La Leche League, its woman-to-woman support can be invaluable for women navigating all these pressures. In her research among members of La Leche League in London and Paris, Charlotte Faircloth found that women would say, 'La Leche League saved my life.'[90]

Supportive networks can be very helpful in dealing with all the judgement and disapproval women have to face, however they feed their babies.

Good Mother Myths and Magical Thinking on Breastfeeding

Out-and-out misogyny explains a lot about why women are so susceptible to being shamed and judged about how they feed their babies. But Good Mother myths play an important role too. Patricia Hamilton has argued that breastfeeding promotion in Britain and Canada (the countries where the mothers she researched lived) is about cultivating certain values among women.

> These efforts promote a vision of mothering that requires intensive efforts, resources and energy to give children the start they 'deserve'. They also idealize a self-responsibilized citizenry, for whom the appropriate amount of breastfeeding is merely one among many consumer choices they are expected to make with no attention paid to the structural constraints that might make another choice more appealing or appropriate.[91]

Andrea Freeman makes a similar point when describing how breastfeeding became valorised in the twentieth century, despite women's feeding options being constrained:

> Cultural beliefs equating nursing with good mothering masked the social and financial realities that drove many Black mothers to alternative feeding methods. Wealthier White women's opportunities to breastfeed became glorified as reflections of choice, not circumstances.[92]

The NCT's *Infant Feeding Message Framework* talks about feeding decisions rather than choices, because the word choice 'implies a range of equal and equally accessible options and this is not the experience of many mothers in the UK'.[93] As I have discussed in this chapter, there are many factors which can narrow and restrict feeding options. Claiming that breastfeeding is in the gift of all women, while ignoring these factors, sets women up to fail.

Women are not only set up to fail on an individual basis. Breastfeeding can be framed as a solution to societal ills such as poverty. In 1985, the UNICEF director James P. Grant described breastfeeding as 'a natural "safety net" against the worst effects of poverty'. He asserted that 'exclusive breastfeeding goes a long way toward cancelling out the health difference between being born into poverty and being born into affluence'.[94] This sweeping claim is still found on UNICEF's website and has been widely quoted elsewhere.[95] One example is a toolkit on infant feeding for English local authorities which claims that increasing breastfeeding rates can 'reduce health inequalities for disadvantaged families'.[96]

There can be an evangelical zeal to these sorts of arguments, just as we see in relation to the crusades about babies' brains. For instance, the psychologist and lactation consultant Kathleen Kendall-Tackett has claimed that 'breastfeeding can make the world a happier and healthier place, one mother and baby at a time'.[97]

But this is yet more magical thinking. As the anthropologist Vanessa Maher argued in the 1990s, exhorting women living in poverty to breastfeed to improve their children's lives puts the burden onto women of 'remedying a situation whose real causes lie in social and political inequalities at both the international and the local level'.[98]

These beliefs also discount the time and effort required for breastfeeding. There is no quarter given for any negative consequences – extended breastfeeding could impact a woman's earning potential for instance. Because of our perceptions of women as givers, the effort and commitment of women who breastfeed are simply taken for granted.

Feeding Rights

The overwhelming evidence that infant feeding can make women miserable has been heard by policymakers. UNICEF UK has said, 'It is time to stop laying the blame for a major public health issue in the laps of individual women and acknowledge the collective responsibility of us all. It is time to change the conversation.'

But nothing in its statement does anything to lessen the burden placed on women or to address the widespread feelings of guilt or shame. If anything, the statement dials up the pressure by calling for the promotion and protection of breastfeeding in all policy areas where breastfeeding is claimed to have an impact, including 'obesity, diabetes and cancer reduction; emotional attachment and subsequent school readiness; improved maternal and child mental health; wellbeing in the workplace; and environmental sustainability'.[99] We have magical thinking to thank for such sweeping claims.

This has led to another double bind. Women are instructed not to feel guilty while simultaneously being guilt-tripped. A good example of this is a statement issued by the Royal College of Midwives following the BBC *Woman's Hour* research discussed earlier: 'Women should not feel guilty if they are struggling to breastfeed their baby or choose not to. While evidence clearly shows that breastfeeding in line with WHO guidance brings optimum benefits for the health of both mother and baby, it is not always possible.'[100]

We must sweep all of this to one side and reframe infant feeding as a feminist issue. As Sheila Kitzinger argued, it should be up to us how we feed our babies, and our breasts belong to us:

There is one powerful argument for artificial [that is, formula] feeding: that the mother herself prefers to do it that way. No other reasons for artificial feeding approach anywhere near the strength of such a statement and if a mother wishes to feed artificially it is her right to do so. She should be able to do this without being made to feel guilty. The choice is hers. Her breasts belong to her.[101]

We need to apply a rights discourse to infant feeding. The psychologists Kate Williams, Ngaire Donaghue and Tim Kurz argue that we must recognise 'the rights of women to adopt the infant-feeding practices that they judge most suitable in their personal circumstances (be this breast-feeding, formula-feeding, or some combination of both)'. They go on to say:

> Feminists need to advocate a woman's right to choose her infant-feeding method in the same way they have championed women's right to real choice in other areas, including occupation, child birth, abortion, and indeed the right to breast-feed. The acceptance of the fact that breast-feeding is not necessarily the best choice for some women – and of the unimpeachable authority of the woman herself to make this decision – is necessary to truly assert that women cannot be guilty for their infant-feeding decisions.[102]

My only issue with this argument is the use of the word 'choice', as we need to bear in mind the ways in which women are constrained personally, economically and socially. But the rest of it – and in particular recognising the 'unimpeachable authority' of women to decide – is spot on.

A central element of this rights discourse must be that women should not be told what to do, treated disrespectfully or touched without permission. Grabbing a woman's breast or speaking to her in a critical or hectoring way are unacceptable. NCT breast-feeding counsellors are trained never to touch a woman's breast or body without consent – this should be standard practice for anyone dealing with women.

Women should not be criticised or shamed for feeding in public or feeding beyond the baby months. The philosopher Fiona Woollard argues that there should be an '*unconditional* moral right to breastfeed in public without social sanction'. In other words, breastfeeding in public should not need to be justified in terms of health or developmental benefits to the child nor should it only be deemed acceptable if certain standards of discretion are met.[103]

Women's decisions must be accepted and supported. Some lip service is currently paid to this, but genuine respect is undermined by the weaselly concept of 'informed choice'. The Royal College of Midwives' statement on infant feeding says that a woman's choice to formula-feed must be respected, *but* only 'after being given appropriate information, advice and support on breastfeeding'.[104] So women cannot simply say, 'No, I don't want to.' Their choice is only accepted if the woman is pressured about breastfeeding first.

A rights discourse must also apply to trans people who have birthed a baby. One qualitative study found that infant feeding can create distressing conflicts with their male or non-binary gender identity. Nevertheless, all the study participants who had not had previous chest masculinisation surgery chose to chestfeed their infants (the term commonly used by trans parents, although the words breastfeeding, nursing and feeding were also used by participants in the study). Similar to the challenges women can face, several experienced 'significant pressure' from healthcare providers, friends or family to chestfeed their babies. Two participants were even advised to chestfeed to protect their legal custody rights as parents.[105] As with women, the 'unimpeachable authority' of trans people to make feeding decisions must be respected.

For these rights to be meaningful, women and trans people who want to breastfeed or chestfeed must be given adequate help and support. This should involve practical guidance, such as positioning the baby at the breast. Sometimes small changes can make all the difference. It is also about identifying issues such as mastitis and tongue tie and finding a way through these. A Cochrane Review concluded that extra support over and above standard maternity care, whether delivered by health professionals or lay/peer supporters, results in women breastfeeding for longer.[106] This support needs to be both practical and emotional, with more honesty about the potential difficulties of breastfeeding and more help on how to overcome problems. Breastfeeding can be difficult, painful, time consuming, inconvenient and overwhelming. We are doing women no favours by sweeping all of this under the carpet and then not providing them with help when they need it.

We also desperately need some well-designed research which examines why some women can't breastfeed. There is a whole host of feeding issues where we just don't have enough knowledge: what is effective in dealing with milk supply problems, what can help with nipple pain and how best to deal with engorgement, mastitis and tongue tie.

Women who want to formula-feed should be given clear and non-judgemental advice on how to do so, particularly relating to making up bottles safely. More guidance and research are needed on combining breast and bottle-feeding, which can be a good option for some women.

We should remain deeply suspicious of the formula companies, ready to exploit any weakness in arguments for breastfeeding. Perhaps it is time for radical action because formula milk is a necessity which every family should be able to access. Amy Brown argues that formula milk should be a generic product, as infant formula brands in the UK and the European Union already have to follow strict regulations on their composition. She rightly rejects the suggestion that is sometimes made that formula should only be available on prescription. This sort of thinking, along with arguments that formula should have large health warnings like a packet of cigarettes, only serves to stigmatise families.[107]

We cannot go on as we are. Women are set up to fail. They simultaneously face pressures to feed in one way but barriers to do so and a lack of support. Because discussions about feeding take place in the context of Good Mother myths, women can conceal their difficulties and feelings. Fear of judgement can put women off seeking help or hide that they are mixing breast and bottle or would like to stop breastfeeding altogether.[108]

Feeding is the site of all the contradictions and pressures on women and mothers – our bodies, our role in society and the clashing currents of commerce, morality, politics and blame. A rights-based approach to feeding would confront all of this head-on.

We also need to call out the misogyny which drives so much of the venom around feeding. This misogyny is fuelled by moral outrage about mothers failing to be givers, whether this is withholding their breasts from babies or from men. However, it is not only directed at mothers of young children but also women who are breastfeeding supporters, who can find themselves being insulted in hyperbolic fashion with terms such as 'breastapo' or 'breastfeeding Nazis'.

Much of this virulence comes from other women. One of the most painful elements of Good Mother myths is how they pit women against each other. Feeding, like birth, is a particularly agonising example of this. At the core of motherdom should be the conviction that compassion is better than censure when we contemplate women's choices and experiences.

5

Attachment Issues

Insensitive mothers have insecure children who grow up to be screwed-up adults. This is a Good Mother myth we have attachment theory to thank for. It has been a potent source of Good Mother myths. For decades, it has been used to prescribe how Good Mothers should behave. More recently, it has been coupled with neuroscience, with directives now laced with threats of damaged brains. And, like neuroscience, attachment theory is deployed to focus attention on the individual relationship between mother and child, rather than the wider environment of relationships and resources children need to thrive.

Attachment theory is presented as scientific truth. But the claims made are often empirically dubious, muddled and shade into magical thinking. It is an excellent example of how research can be guided by unthinking assumptions, such as ignoring children's network of relationships. It is also a cautionary tale of how research can be distorted and exploited by advocacy groups and social entrepreneurs who, in the words of the social scientist Robbie Duschinsky, have circulated versions of attachment theory that 'in important ways run contrary to available empirical evidence'.[1]

Attachment Theory Started with Mother Love

As we shall see, attachment theory now has global influence, but it is an Anglo-American creation, conceived by John Bowlby and Mary Ainsworth. Ainsworth enters the story later, so we shall begin with Bowlby. Born in 1907, Bowlby's experience of maternal care was typical of an upper-middle-class British child of his era; he was mostly looked after by a nanny and nursemaids. Bowlby's mother would call into the nursery in the morning, and then Bowlby and his siblings only saw her again on a visit to the drawing room between 5 and 6 pm.

A nursemaid named Minnie cared for Bowlby on a daily basis until he was four, when she left the Bowlby household. Bowlby never discussed her departure directly, although he would write in 1958 that the loss of a loving nanny can be almost as tragic as the loss of a mother.[2] Bowlby's father was away for almost five years during the First World War and only visited his family a handful of times. When his father finally returned home in 1918, Bowlby was sent to boarding school. He was aged ten at the time and was only allowed home during school holidays. On one of these visits, he saw his godfather drop down dead in front of him during a game of football.[3]

We can speculate how far Bowlby's childhood experiences of separation and emotional deprivation influenced his work as a psychiatrist, psychologist and psychoanalyst. According to his wife, Ursula, Bowlby himself wasn't much interested in introspection. In a letter to the psychologist Robert Karen, she commented, 'John wasn't curious about people, about "how they ticked," and he was very *in*curious about himself.'[4]

What is clear is that the intellectual influence of Sigmund Freud and prevailing cultural beliefs about mothers are two central pillars of Bowlby's work. Freud's 1938 claim that mothers are 'unique, without parallel, laid down unalterably for a whole lifetime as the first and strongest love-object and as the prototype of all later love relations' was quoted by both Bowlby and Ainsworth in different papers.[5] Throughout his long career, Bowlby's background assumption, to use Helen Longino's term, was that mothers shape their children, for good or for ill.

Bowlby's first great work of influence was *Child Care and the Growth of Love* published in 1953, which was based on a report he had written for the World Health Organization on the welfare of homeless children. Bowlby famously declared: 'Mother-love in infancy and childhood is as important for mental health as are vitamins and proteins for physical health.' Bowlby asserted that it is 'essential' for a child's future mental health to 'experience a warm, intimate, and continuous relationship with his mother (or permanent mother-substitute – one person who steadily "mothers" him) in which both find satisfaction and enjoyment'.[6]

Bowlby's arguments quickly took hold.[7] For instance, the 1948 edition of *Housewife Baby Book*, published by *Housewife Magazine,* includes a chapter entitled 'Nurse, Nanny or Mother's Help' which recommends getting paid assistance after the birth of a baby. The book advises that this is worth the expense: 'The cost is undoubtedly very high, but even the temporary services of a really well-trained nurse for, say, three or four months may make such a difference to an over-strained mother that it is sometimes worthwhile to dip into a little capital to obtain it.'[8]

In the 1955 edition, published less than a decade later, the advice is very different. The chapter has been retitled 'Substitute Mothers' and it begins:

> Recent researches have demonstrated very clearly the immense importance to a baby of the constant presence of a mother during the early years of life. For the first few months it is the mother only who feeds and tends him and in this way he learns to recognise the feel of her arms and the sound of her voice, which gradually bring that sense of security which is the aim of all true mothercraft to produce.

The new edition of *Housewife Baby Book* advises that substitute mothers are permissible in certain circumstances *after* the first few months, although only if they are 'really good'. The mother should remain her baby's 'main source of physical and mental comfort'.[9] The over-strained mother who could do with some help has fallen out of view.

Although Bowlby's work was popular, his evidence and conclusions were comprehensively challenged in the years that followed the publication of *Child Care and the Growth of Love*. 'None of Bowlby's references offers satisfactory evidence that maternal deprivation is harmful for the young infant,' the American psychologist Lawrence Casler concluded in 1961.[10]

In response to these arguments, the World Health Organization published *Deprivation of Maternal Care: A Reassessment of Its Effects* in 1962.[11] All the chapters in this book, with the exception of a piece written by Mary Ainsworth, highlighted the lack of evidence in support of Bowlby's views. Barbara Wootton, a distinguished social scientist, wrote, 'Whatever the future may show, reference in the present state of knowledge to the "permanent," "irreversible" or "irreparable" damage due to separation is reckless and unjustified.'[12]

Key shortcomings identified in all the critiques were that studies were carried out among small (sometimes tiny) groups of children, many of the studies referred to the same group of children, there were no 'control' groups to compare the children with and most of the research was done with children from institutions or hospitals. As with neuroscience narratives today, extreme examples of deprivation were used to make wider generalisations about families.

Arguably the most serious flaw in Bowlby's work was the bundling together of a range of problems, such as being separated from the entire family, into the category of 'maternal care and love'. He did not distinguish between separation from the mother and wider deprivation. His foundational belief was that everything could, and should, be traced back to mothers.

Bowlby's faith in the importance of mother love was unshaken by criticism and remained central to his work. In 1969 he published *Attachment*, the first volume of his trilogy *Attachment and Loss*. Bowlby defined attachment behaviour 'as seeking and maintaining proximity to another individual'. He argued that this is innate because of what he called the 'environment of evolutionary adaptedness' – infants who were biologically predisposed to stay close to their mothers were less likely to be killed by predators. By claiming that attachment has a biological basis, Bowlby drew upon the moral authority of 'nature'. A picture at the front of *Attachment*, used as the cover of the paperback edition, evokes 'natural' and 'primitive' tropes by depicting a naked mother from the Amazon basin carrying an infant on her hip and a container of water on her head.

In the book, Bowlby outlined the dynamics of attachment, explaining how infants' attachment behaviours can draw their carers to them (for example, through crying, smiling and babbling) and also keep them nearby (for example, through clinging and, when the baby is older, following). These behaviours encourage caregivers to provide protection, comfort and support. Many factors can activate attachment behaviours, for instance when babies are hungry, tired, cold or unwell or the caregiver is leaving.

This was all written in terms of mothers and babies (who Bowlby refers to as 'he' without fail). There is a short section towards the end of the book where Bowlby discussed alternative attachment figures. He stated that it is 'abundantly clear' that a child's principal attachment figure can be someone other than a mother but, echoing what he had written earlier, only if this person is 'a mother-substitute [who] behaves in a mothering way towards a child'.[13] This was a conviction he held throughout his life. In the last interview he gave before his death in 1990, he said that in order to grow up 'healthy, happy, self-reliant, and confident' children need their mother (or a mother figure) to be their principal caregiver.[14]

Bowlby never acknowledged or examined the assumptions that underpinned his work. He was selective in the animal research he drew upon, focusing on patterns of behaviour which conformed to his ideal of constant and attentive maternal care. However, there is an enormous amount of variation in behaviour between animals, even within the same species. Recall the anthropologist Sarah Hrdy's description of continuous-care-and-contact mothering as 'a last resort' for primates who lack safe and available alternatives.[15]

Bowlby was very much a creature of his time. He equated healthy adult development with heterosexual marriage and having children. In a lecture given in 1986, he remarked that people with affectionate and responsive parents 'are far more likely than those who come from less stable and supportive homes to make stable marriages and to provide their children with the same favourable conditions for healthy development that they enjoyed themselves'.[16] For most of his life, homosexuality was illegal in the UK; it was only decriminalised in 1967 in England and Wales, in 1981 in Scotland and 1982 in Northern Ireland. In *Attachment*, he quoted the psychologist Harry Harlow's findings from his notorious experiments on primates: 'Heterosexual behaviour is greatly influenced by early experience, and the failure of infants to form effective infant–infant affectional relations delays or destroys adequate adult heterosexual behaviour.'[17]

Like Freud, who wrote that women 'stand for the interests of the family and sexual life' but have 'little aptitude' for what he called the work of civilisation, Bowlby believed that men and women have different roles and needs.[18] He was opposed to mothers working, saying a year before his death: 'I do not think it's a good idea. I mean women go out to work and make some fiddly little bit of gadgetry which has no particular social value, and children are looked after in indifferent day nurseries.'[19] Robbie Duschinsky recounts that Bowlby made 'harsh and mocking remarks' about his feminist critics, for instance claiming in an interview that professional women had a vested interest in criticising his theories of maternal deprivation because they had neglected their own families.[20] Ainsworth, who deeply regretted not having children herself, was more considered. Towards the end of her long career, she wrote:

Had I myself had the children for whom I vainly longed, I like to believe that I could have arrived at some satisfactory combination of mothering and a career, but I do not believe that there is any universal, easy, ready-made solution to the problem.[21]

Bowlby's work was a mirror reflecting, but also magnifying, beliefs about the role of women. The norm of the male bread-winner and female homemaker was reasserted in the UK and US following the end of the Second World War. High levels of participation in the wartime workforce by women were reversed and public funding for day care ended. Working mothers (and there continued to be working mothers) relied once again on what the historian Helen McCarthy describes as 'low-cost informal arrangements within the family and community'.[22]

As with today's neuroscience advocates, there was an evangelical slant to Bowlby's work. The anthropologist Robert LeVine describes him as a reformer as well as a scientist and argues that attachment research should be 'seen as part of a twentieth century moral campaign to change childcare in Britain and America'.[23] Children were routinely separated from their families, for instance when ill in hospital. It was thanks to Bowlby that the tide of professional opinion turned firmly against this (although as late as the 1980s only half of English hospitals offered parents unrestricted visiting).[24]

As Bowlby said himself: 'I'm the kind of person who identifies a typhoid bacillus and says, "Look, if you let typhoid bacilli get into the water supply, there'll be trouble." That's been my job in life.' It was his hope that the lasting value of attachment theory would be 'the light it throws on the conditions most likely to promote healthy personality development. Only when those conditions are clear beyond doubt will parents know what is best for their children and will communities be willing to help them provide it.'[25]

But blurring the lines between scientific enquiry and advocacy can be dangerous. One tragic outcome of Bowlby's influence was his strong support for very early adoption: '[It's] in the interests of the adopted baby's mental health for him to be adopted soon after birth.'[26] This shaped adoption policies in favour of a 'clean break' and led to babies being forcibly taken from their mothers immediately or soon after they had given birth.[27]

Mary Ainsworth to the Rescue

It was pure chance that Mary Ainsworth and Bowlby ever met. If they had not, attachment theory would have been a much less potent force, and it is unlikely that we would still be talking about it today. Attachment researchers recognise Ainsworth as the co-founder of attachment theory, but some popularisers of attachment thinking ignore her. For instance, a report called *Baby Bonds*, which we shall consider later in this chapter, describes Bowlby as 'the founder of attachment theory' and does not mention Ainsworth at all.[28]

In her excellent history of attachment theory, the historian of science Marga Vicedo relates how Bowlby's work continued to be criticised in the 1960s and 1970s.[29] A particularly serious challenge was made by James Robertson because he was Bowlby's long-time collaborator who provided, in Bowlby's own words, the 'main data' he had drawn upon in the 1969 edition of *Attachment*. Robertson was a social worker who had conducted observational research on the impact of children being separated from their families in hospitals. In the acknowledgements of *Attachment*, Bowlby said that 'my debt to him is immense'.[30] In a 1971 paper co-authored with his wife, Robertson echoed earlier criticisms of how Bowlby had extrapolated data from hospitals to everyday separations from mothers: 'Bowlby, without adducing non-institutional data, has generalized Robertson's concept of protest, despair, and denial beyond the context from which it was derived . . . Our findings do not support Bowlby's generalizations about the responses of young children to loss of the mother.'[31]

Ainsworth's pioneering research filled the vacuum left by Robertson. In Vicedo's words, she 'provided much-needed empirical backing for his theoretical views'.[32] Ainsworth's and Bowlby's paths happened to cross because she moved to London in 1950 with her husband so he could finish his graduate degree at University College. She gave up her job as a psychologist at the University of Toronto and was unable to find another position in advance of their move. She later recalled: 'Upon arrival in London, I immediately cast about for a job.' She was alerted to an advert in the *Times Educational Supplement* 'for a job that seemed precisely suited to my qualifications. It was for a research position at the Tavistock Clinic in an investigation, directed by Dr John Bowlby, into the effect on personality development of separation from the mother in early childhood.'[33]

And so began Ainsworth's and Bowlby's long and fruitful collaboration. A paper she co-authored with Bowlby in 1956 was the first instance of either of them using the word 'attachment' in their work.[34] Ainsworth made several fundamental contributions to attachment theory. She formulated the concept of the attachment figure as a secure base from which infants explore the world, distinguishing between exploratory and attachment behaviours.[35] She developed attachment classifications (initially just secure and insecure). She linked maternal sensitivity with secure attachments, which we will explore in more detail later in this chapter.[36] But arguably her most influential contribution was the invention of the Strange Situation test. This allowed attachment status to be tested in a laboratory setting in twenty minutes and spawned a whole body of research. As Robert Karen notes, by the early 1980s, universities all over the US were populated with attachment scholars.[37]

Ainsworth left London in 1954 and sailed to Uganda with her husband, who was starting a job as a research psychologist in Kampala. There, she undertook what she described as 'a naturalistic study' of mother–infant interaction with twenty-eight babies and twenty-six mothers (there were two sets of twins).[38] While this work has been presented as independently confirming Bowlby's theories (and as evidence of its cross-cultural applicability), Vicedo convincingly argues that Ainsworth's collaboration with Bowlby influenced how she interpreted her data, which she did not actually write up until almost a decade after doing the fieldwork.

In her study, Ainsworth observed that specific patterns of maternal care were correlated with certain infant behaviours. Like Bowlby, her foundational assumption was that maternal care was the cause of these behaviours. Ainsworth failed to apply the basic tenet of scientific enquiry that correlation is not causation. In addition, her analysis did not, as Vicedo points out, attempt to take into account any other factors that could influence a child's behaviour. For instance, she did not consider that some of the babies were taken care of by several people and not just their mothers.[39]

Ainsworth then followed her husband to Baltimore in 1955 (the marriage broke up five years later which she subsequently described as a 'personal disaster'). She was offered a position at Johns Hopkins University and in 1963 began work on her famous Baltimore study. Twenty-six babies from White, middle-class families, were recruited through paediatricians in private practice. These babies were visited at home every three weeks from three to fifty-four weeks of age. At around the age of one, twenty-three of the babies (one baby from the original sample was too old and another two were ill) took part in a laboratory assessment which was named the Strange Situation.[40] Several influential papers on the Baltimore study appeared over the next decade, with the first coming out in 1969.[41] A book summarising the findings was published in 1978.[42]

The Strange Situation test, which Ainsworth devised with her colleague Barbara Wittig, involves a series of episodes in which the baby plays in a laboratory room. At first, both the parent and a researcher are present. The parent leaves the room and then returns for a brief period of play and then both the parent and researcher leave. The baby is left alone for about three minutes and then the researcher returns. After another three minutes, the parent returns. It is the baby's interaction with their parent at this point which is assessed to determine their attachment status.

In the Baltimore study, three main groups were identified and broken down further into subgroups (the subgroups were tiny, some only had one or two babies in them). Babies who sought contact with their mothers during the reunion were classified as having a secure attachment. Babies who showed little desire to seek proximity to their mother and tended to avoid her, for instance by turning away, were labelled 'avoidant'. A third group of babies (four in total) were described as 'heterogeneous', bracketed together on the basis of what was 'loosely specified as "maladaptive behaviour"'. Their attachment was later described as 'resistant'.

These groups were then compared with classifications made on all the home visits in the final three months of the baby's first year. The home and laboratory classifications were found to be significantly related, with the common factor being 'the degree of sensitivity the mother showed to the baby's signals, in noticing them, interpreting them accurately, and in responding to them promptly and appropriately'. Mothers of secure babies were significantly more sensitive than mothers of avoidant and resistant babies. However, in the three secure subgroups, only one group (of nine babies) showed high levels of sensitivity, while the other two groups (of four babies in total) were 'moderately' or 'inconsistently' sensitive. Within the 'resistant' group, there were two babies who behaved similarly in the Strange Situation procedure, but the behaviour of their mothers in the home setting was 'disparate'.[43]

These attachment classifications are quite an edifice to build on the basis of only twenty-three babies (there were other samples used in the development of the Strange Situation procedure, but this was the only sample where behaviour in the laboratory could be related back to home behaviour). Remember the law of small numbers which was discussed in Chapter 2; the fewer times you roll the dice, the more likely that the patterns you find do not accurately reflect reality. Ainsworth herself was well aware that her Baltimore sample size was very small and that the study needed to be replicated. She wrote in 1971 that 'adequate validation of our strange-situation procedure as a test of infant-mother attachment will require a series of replicatory studies with different samples' and that 'much more research is obviously required both to replicate and confirm our findings'.[44] However, when she applied for funding to do just that, she was repeatedly turned down.[45]

The Baltimore study was subject to a detailed critique in a 1984 paper written by a group of researchers led by developmental psychologist Michael Lamb (who was also one of the academics who took apart bonding theory). It highlighted the small sample size, drily noting that twenty-three babies is 'hardly an adequate data base for generating an exhaustive and "species-typical" set of categories'. Another problem flagged was that firm conclusions had been drawn from small differences. For instance, it was reported that mothers of avoidant infants use 'forcible physical interventions' more frequently than mothers of secure infants, even though there was only a difference of 0.7 physical interactions in a four-hour visit.

The paper also pointed out that the Strange Situation test rests on an assumption that differences in the way infants behave in a laboratory test are related to differences in the nature of their relationship with a caregiver. A clear logical flaw in the Baltimore study was that although babies in the 'avoidant' and 'resistant' groups behaved very differently in the Strange Situation test, there were no clear differences between the mothers. This meant that it is not then possible to infer that behaviour in the Strange Situation 'is lawfully determined by prior patterns of infant-mother interaction'.

These issues, together with shortcomings such as a failure to check the reliability of researchers observing in-home, resulted in a highly critical verdict on the Baltimore study:

This project must be viewed *solely* [original emphasis] as a hypothesis-generating pilot study – not as a hypothesis-testing investigation. The findings can only obtain generalizability when replicated in independent studies in which bias is controlled and a priori predictions are tested and verified.[46]

Lamb's paper was met with horror by attachment theorists (Ainsworth herself maintained 'a stony public silence' according to Karen), and they refused to submit the usual comments or rebuttals to the journal that published it.[47] There were personal reasons for this. Ainsworth was held in great affection and regard by other attachment researchers. Inge Bretherton, a leading attachment researcher who was one of Ainsworth's students, described her as an 'exacting and caring' mentor who 'conveyed a deep personal interest' in her doctoral studies and provided 'unusually generous help' to other researchers in the field.[48] But another likely factor was that by this point attachment research had gained considerable traction, thanks to the Strange Situation test. With numerous studies conducted and underway, it might be better not to peer under the bonnet too closely.

So despite its tiny sample size and serious flaws, Ainsworth's study of twenty-three babies has been extraordinarily influential and is still referenced as evidence, both in the academic and policy literature. For instance, a 2024 research review on neuro-development and mental health in early life cites Ainsworth's 1978 book *Patterns of Attachment: A Psychological Study of the Strange Situation* in support of the claim 'healthy attachment, an established predictor of child development, emphasises consistent responsive parental behaviour'.[49]

It is a classic example of how academic work that is continually cited eventually becomes seminal and, as David Wastell and Sue White put it, 'contestable findings can become rewritten as fundamental truths'.[50]

Being Sensitive about Sensitivity

The Baltimore study has arguably had its strongest impact on contemporary Good Mother myths (as well as policy prescriptions) by promoting the belief that sensitive care leads to a secure attachment. 'Responsive caregiving', which requires caregivers to be 'sensitive and responsive to the child's cues', is a core component of the Nurturing Care Framework which has been adopted by global bodies such as the World Health Organization.[51] The hegemony of sensitivity has been buttressed by brain claims. For instance, the First 1001 Days Movement has claimed 'after birth, sensitive, responsive interactions and healthy relationships with caregivers are particularly important for early brain development'.[52]

But what is actually meant by sensitivity? At the heart of Ainsworth's definition is the effacement of the mother's needs and wishes. The highly sensitive mother is 'exquisitely attuned' to the baby's signals and responds to them 'promptly and appropriately'. By contrast, the highly insensitive mother is 'geared almost exclusively to her own wishes, moods and activity'.[53] Bowlby similarly defined sensitivity in terms of constant availability to the baby:

> It is characteristic of a mother whose infant will develop securely that she is continuously monitoring her infant's state and, as and when he signals wanting attention, she registers his signals and acts accordingly. By contrast, the mother of an infant later found to be anxiously attached is likely to monitor her infant's state only sporadically and, when she does notice his signals, to respond tardily and/or inappropriately.[54]

There is no acknowledgement or allowance that mothers may have other commitments or concerns, such as older children or work. Bowlby had long held the view that nothing less than constant attention would do. In a pamphlet for mothers written in 1958, he advised:

By all means let a mother take a half-day off, or even an occasional whole day, but anything longer needs careful management . . . It is essential to leave him in the care of one person, who will be a mother-figure to him while you are away. If you can follow this plan, you will be providing for your child the essential security which he needs in his early years, the benefits of which both of you will reap in the years to come.[55]

Sweeping claims continue to be made about the importance of sensitivity. An influential report, entitled *Baby Bonds*, published by the Sutton Trust, a charity which aims to improve social mobility through education, states that 'the overwhelming finding in our review is that warm, sensitive, and responsive care, from both mothers and fathers, builds secure attachment.'[56] Note the use of attachment in the singular. This is muddled thinking because the term 'attachment' relates to a relationship between a child and caregiver – it is not a label that is used to describe an individual child. We shall see several more examples of this from attachment evangelists.

Even worse is the claim in a report written by the Social Mobility Commission, a body created by the UK government, that 'the more sensitive and responsive, and warm the relationship, the more secure the attachment'.[57] Ainsworth explicitly rejected classifying attachment in terms of degrees of security, and attachment research does not measure strengths of attachment.[58] The report writers unthinkingly, and without a shred of evidence, parrot the current orthodoxy of the more the better.

To put it plainly, these attachment advocates are distorting the evidence. Ainsworth's finding of a strong relationship between maternal sensitivity and attachment security has not been replicated in other research. A 1997 meta-analysis carried out by attachment researchers Marianne De Wolff and Marinus H. van IJzendoorn looked at how attachment status relates to maternal sensitivity. They found only a modest relationship between sensitivity and attachment as measured in the Strange Situation (there was a combined effect size of 0.24 in twenty-one studies with 1,099 babies). They concluded that 'sensitivity cannot be considered to be the exclusive and most important factor in the development of attachment.'[59]

There are some situations where little or no relationship has been found between sensitivity and attachment classification. In the case of fathers, a meta-analysis of sixteen studies with a combined sample size of 1,355 found that paternal sensitivity and attachment were only weakly correlated (the effect size was 0.12).[60] In an unusually large attachment study (the sample size was 1,153), there was no relationship between maternal sensitivity and attachment security for infants in high-quality childcare, although there was for infants in low-quality care (quality of care was assessed by observing caregivers on behaviours such as responding to distress, physical care, and talking and reading to children).[61]

There are many factors which impact on children's relationships with their parents. A meta-analysis of fifty-five studies of 4,792 children found that disorganised attachment, a fourth category of attachment first proposed by Mary Main and Judith Solomon in 1986, is as likely to be found in children from families experiencing five or more socioeconomic risk factors (such as low income and single parenthood) as infants who had been maltreated.[62]

An obsession with maternal sensitivity leads us down blind alleys. This is illustrated by the Minding the Baby® programme (and yes, it does have a registered trademark). This is an intensive home visiting programme aimed at young mothers and children living in adverse socioeconomic circumstances. A randomised, controlled trial in the UK among 148 first-time mothers aged under twenty-six to assess the impact of the programme chose maternal sensitivity as the primary outcome and found no difference between the control and treatment groups.[63]

In research terms, sensitivity is a vague and nebulous concept. There is no consensus among attachment researchers on how to measure it. A systematic review conducted by two researchers from Leiden University's Centre for Child and Family Studies unearthed fifty different observational instruments used to measure parental sensitivity in early childhood. The review observed that studies on the components of sensitivity are 'surprisingly rare'. Of the eight sensitivity scales that the review looked at in detail, only two were underpinned by a clear theoretical framework.[64]

However, 'sensitivity' as a concept is clearly rooted in Good Mother myths which reflect cultural ideals of Western, White, middle-class mothering. Good Mothers are constantly available to their children and interact with them continuously to cultivate their emotional and cognitive development. As Robert LeVine points out, sensitivity involves 'moral judgements specific to the Anglo-American cultural ideology of parent-child interaction that became influential in the mid twentieth century and has remained so'.[65]

We can see this in the Maternal Behaviour Q-Sort, one of the better-known ways of measuring sensitivity.[66] It is 'sensitive' to point out interesting things to the baby, provide age-appropriate toys and to talk to the baby throughout the assessment. The 'insensitive' mother decides on naptimes convenient for her and stops interacting with the baby if the telephone rings or to talk to a visitor. Most bizarrely of all, the insensitive mother 'uses sibling or television' to keep the baby entertained. I think we can all agree that equating a baby's sibling with a television is pretty insensitive.

In many cultures, early caregiving is characterised by extensive bodily contact and little face-to-face or vocal interaction. In a study of twenty-eight Gusii babies, the babies were observed to be in constant bodily contact with a caregiver. Gusii caregivers were found to respond quickly to a baby's cries with breastfeeding or gentle jiggling, but infrequently to the baby's babbling or eye contact compared with a sample of American mothers.[67] Which pattern of caregiving should we regard as sensitive – the Gusii, the American or both of them?

Some attachment researchers have turned their attention away from sensitivity.[68] They have suggested focusing instead on the concept of 'secure base provision'. This is about providing a 'safe haven' when the baby's attachment system is activated (that is, when they are tired, hungry, afraid or in pain) and enabling them to explore when they are calm. In a study of eighty-three babies of low-income American mothers, 'secure base provision' was assessed in terms of maternal responses to the baby during both crying and non-crying episodes. 'Secure base provision' was judged to be present when at least half of crying episodes ended in chest-to-chest soothing and when in non-crying episodes there was 'calm, regulating connectedness (e.g., being available for eye contact without actively seeking eye contact, carrying the infant on the hip during daily tasks)'.

The study found that maternal sensitivity did not predict infant attachment, but 'secure base provision' did. Susan S. Woodhouse, the lead researcher, observed 'responses to infant fussing were not especially important – it was picking up and soothing the baby when the infant cried that made a difference. The baby came to see the parent as a secure base who, on average, could be counted on to be there when it really mattered.'[69]

'Secure base provision' – someone a child can generally count on when it matters – feels to me like a more realistic, humane and respectful way of thinking about attachment. Hopefully it will, as the researchers suggest, open up new avenues of research and practice.[70]

We must bring to an end moralising about maternal sensitivity, as well as educational programmes which instruct women on how to mother 'sensitively'. In their paper ' "Poor Brain Development" in the Global South? Challenging the Science of Early Childhood Interventions', the anthropologist Gabriel Scheidecker and his fellow authors question the value of providing unsolicited training to parents in the Global South on how to interact with their children. Instead, 'sensitive responsiveness' should be directed towards understanding what interventions families and communities actually want.[71]

The Internal Working (or Non-working?) Model

Another element of attachment theory that rests on shaky assumptions is the so-called 'internal working model'. It purports to explain how attachment works its magic (or malice) over time. The children's charity NSPCC said in a report on vulnerable babies (and note the reference to a single caregiver):

> Attachment patterns develop in early relationships and inter-action with the primary caregiver, which lead to the development of 'internal working models' that then inform the way an individual feels about him/her self and relations with other people.[72]

However, the concept is, to be charitable, a working hypothesis which needs a lot of ironing out. In a lecture given in 1980, Bowlby acknowledged that understanding of internal working models was 'still scanty'.[73] Things have not moved on a great deal since then. As one attachment researcher puts it, 'the field needs greater theoretical development of the IWM [internal working model] concept'.[74] The lack of a firm theoretical underpinning is illustrated by the tendency of researchers to cite Bowlby's work, written decades ago, to evidence the concept.

A key conundrum is explaining how the internal working model develops when a child has more than one attachment. Attachment researchers Carollee Howes and Susan Spieker identify three different potential theories. There is the hierarchical approach, where the child's representation of the most significant caregiver is the most influential. There is the integrative theory, where the child integrates all attachment relationships into a single representation. Finally, there is the independent theory, in which the different representations are independent both in quality and their influence on development.[75] We just don't know which of these explanations is most valid. Alan Sroufe, who led the famous Minnesota Longitudinal Study among parents and children, which started in 1975, writes that 'to date I know of no studies of this truly critical question'.[76]

Nevertheless, it seems to be the hierarchical theory that holds sway in popular thinking; the NSPCC definition quoted earlier refers to the primary caregiver (although it also, confusingly, refers to models in the plural). However, it is the least plausible of all the theories. Just as very young children can understand that dogs go woof but goldfish don't, they learn that not every person or relationship is alike. As the cognitive psychologist Steven Pinker puts it, relationships with parents, siblings and peers differ and 'the trillion-synapse human brain is hardly short of the computational power it would take to keep each one in a separate mental account'.[77] It also doesn't make much evolutionary sense for children to have an inflexible view of relationships shaped by one caregiver. It is hard to see how this would have increased their chances of survival.

But flimsy as it may be, the concept of the internal working model persists because of deep-seated cultural beliefs about the power of mothers to permanently mould their children.

The Influence of Early Attachments

Perhaps the biggest gulf between the work of attachment researchers, including Bowlby himself, and popularisers of attachment theory is the significance of early attachments. Attachment evangelists portray secure early attachments as providing long-lasting benefits for individual children. The Sutton Trust's report *Baby Bonds* claims that 'an early secure attachment appears to have a lasting positive effect on children's outcomes'.[78] The apparent dangers of insecure attachments are then used to justify interference in the everyday lives of mothers and babies.

There are some who question the very basic assumption at the heart of attachment theory; that universal secure attachment is something we should be aiming for in the first place. Robbie

Duschinsky observes that attachment researchers today commonly believe that attachment security is not necessarily always best in both the short and the long term.[79] The psychologist Elizabeth Meins, who Duschinsky describes as one of the UK's leading attachment researchers in the 1990s and 2000s, has made this point particularly strongly:

> The belief that making all toddlers securely attached will have knock-on positive effects for future generations is patently incorrect . . . Different types of attachment simply reflect the kind of individual differences you'd expect to see in any aspect of children's early development. People are perfectly happy with variation in toddlers' height, weight and ability to walk and talk, but don't want variation in attachment relationships.[80]

This is in stark contrast to popular portrayals of attachment theory. Insecure attachments are misleadingly equated with inevitably bad outcomes for children. The Sutton Trust's *Baby Bonds* report recommends 'parent training' and a basket of other interventions to promote a secure attachment (attachment is referred to in the singular throughout the report). These interventions 'may be able to prevent problems and reduce the need for costly health, education, social and criminal justice services'.[81]

The Wave Trust, an influential player in early intervention policy in the UK, goes even further.[82] In a report funded by the UK government, it put forward a recommendation which is both chilling and absurd: a universal assessment when babies are three to four months old to assess the quality of the parent (note the singular) and infant interaction. This is in order to 'identify need for additional support to promote parental sensitive responsiveness'. In the appendix of the report, the pretence that this assessment could involve either parent is ditched: 'Without assessing every mother-infant dyad, attachment difficulties would be missed at this crucial early stage.'[83]

In their zeal to catch insecure attachments as early as possible, the report writers seem unaware that a central premise of attachment theory is that attachments do not usually develop until six months at least.[84] Indeed, a consensus statement produced by seventy attachment researchers states that 'it is currently not advisable to assess children's attachment quality until the age of about one'.

This consensus statement also warns against the dangers of using attachment theory at an individual level: 'The effects [of secure attachment] are not of a size to imply that a child's future development can be predicted with confidence solely from assessments of attachment security.'[85] This echoes warnings from an earlier paper produced by forty-three attachment researchers, including some of the best-known names in the field, such as Alan Sroufe, Mary Main and Judith Solomon. The paper criticised the 'myths or exaggerations regarding disorganised attachment without support from research evidence'. It points out that disorganised attachment is not a definitive assessment at an individual level, nor does it reliably indicate child maltreatment or predict pathology: 'Research at the *group* level [my emphasis] has established disorganized infant attachment as a small-moderate predictor for the development of social and behaviour problems.'[86]

Bowlby himself, guided by his clinical experience, was optimistic about the potential of people's ability to overcome early adversity:

> Since the course of subsequent development is not fixed, changes in the way a child is treated can shift his pathway in either a more favourable direction or a less favourable one. Although the capacity for developmental change diminishes with age, change continues throughout the life cycle so that changes for better or for worse are always possible.[87]

Alan Sroufe makes it clear that 'change, as well as continuity, is central to the theory'. Attachment classifications can and do change over time and the longer the period between measurements, the less stability there is. In periods longer than fifteen years, there is no significant stability at all.[88] In Sroufe's Minnesota study, factors associated with a change in attachment status included family life stress and social support.[89] After decades of attachment research, Sroufe concludes, 'We can put aside debates about whether early experience or later experience, or parenting or peer experiences, are more important. We know they are all important and we know they work together to shape development.'[90]

The Value of Multiple Attachments

It's easier to research the relationship with only one parent. But the focus on one caregiver is largely ideological. Bowlby and Ainsworth viewed the world through the prism of mothers and babies. As we have seen, Bowlby recognised that infants could have more than one attachment figure, but he maintained that principal attachment figures must behave 'in a mothering way'.[91] Because of their focus on mothers, Bowlby and Ainsworth, as Magda Vicedo points out, never studied any of the other people who take care of children, such as fathers, grandparents, aunts, uncles or siblings.[92]

There has since been some limited research on the impact of different attachments. For instance, a US study of eighty-six two-parent families assessed children's attachment status with their mother and father using the Strange Situation test at the age of fifteen months. The children's behaviour was subsequently rated by teachers at the age of six and a half and then by mothers, fathers and the children themselves at the age of eight. Children with insecure attachments with both parents when they were infants were most likely to have later behavioural issues according to the parents, teachers and children. Having secure attachments with both parents did not seem to add a protective effect beyond security with just one.[93]

Attachment thinking in its most simplistic form ignores these nuances. Popular writing about attachment tends to talk about 'the primary caregiver' (for which read 'mother'). So, for instance, the Wave Trust report we encountered earlier claims: 'With the security of knowing that the primary caregiver is emotionally available, the child grows in confidence to explore the surrounding world, including the learning opportunities of nursery and school.' This report repeatedly talks about attachment in the singular and also makes unscientific claims about brains: 'Good quality relationships and secure attachment enable a growing brain to become efficient.'[94]

Sarah Hrdy argues it would be better to evaluate attachment in terms of how secure a child is in relation to all their caregivers. 'Measuring attachment this way might help explain why even children whose relations with their mother suggest they are at extreme risk manage to do fine because of the interventions of a committed father, an older sibling, or a there-when-you-need-her grandmother.'[95] One group of researchers have proposed a 'Received Sensitivity Scale' to capture the sensitivity experienced from all sources in cultural contexts where simultaneous multiple caregiving is common.[96]

We have seen in the first chapter how caregiving has been shared throughout human history to maximise women's productivity and fertility. This also brings obvious benefits to children. Having several attachment relationships provides children with more sources of comfort and protection. This is a sensible risk-minimisation strategy in case children lose important attachment figures (for most of human history, death rates have been high).[97]

Sarah Hrdy suggests that awareness of diverse perspectives from early in life can make a child more empathetic and enrich their understanding of the emotional states of other people.[98] The developmental psychologist and philosopher Alison Gopnik argues that having different caregivers ensures children are exposed to a wide variety of information and approaches, enabling humans to thrive in a constantly changing world.[99] Bowlby's insistence on 'the absolute need of infants and toddlers for the continuous care of their mothers' fails to take any of this into account.[100]

Putting Attachment Theory in its Place

Despite the many flaws in attachment theory, particularly in its crudest form, it has been enormously influential. One of the reasons why the idea of 'attachment' continues to have such currency is because of 'attachment parenting'. This term was coined in the 1980s by the paediatrician William Sears and his wife Martha, who have published more than forty books on parenting and pregnancy.[101] 'Attachment parenting' involves constant physical contact, breastfeeding, wearing babies in a sling and bed-sharing. In *The Attachment Parenting Book*, the Sears claim that 'attachment parenting' is 'what parents would do naturally without the influence of "experts"'.

The Sears deploy science along with nature, with sections entitled 'Science Says' which make claims such as 'AP babies' are likely to be smarter and have enhanced motor development.[102] Patricia Hamilton highlights the contradiction that 'an imagined Africa defined by its "natural" style of childrearing' is then 'translated into rational, scientifically supported parenting advice by the likes of the Sears'.[103]

Attachment thinking has influenced policymakers as well as parents throughout the globe. As we have seen, the promotion of a specific type of parenting throughout the developing world has been mandated on the basis of attachment theory.

Good Mother myths based on attachment thinking have even found their way to Iceland, the poster child for gender equality, which consistently ranks top of the World Economic Forum's annual Global Gender Gap Report.[104] When social scientist Sunna Símonardóttir analysed Icelandic public health websites, she found that attachment theory has 'become a part of the landscape of contemporary childcare advice and knowledge . . . Certain "truths" become scientifically sanctioned and reasonable, while conflicting discourses are made to seem inappropriate or even unnatural.' These websites promote 'classic ideas about the primacy of the mother', with 'little effort' to include fathers. Behaviour and emotions are prescribed; mothers are supposed to be 'happy, calm, and content' and to 'direct all their physical and emotional capacities at their children'.[105]

Attachment thinking holds particular sway in the UK. The academics Val Gillies, Rosalind Edwards and Nicola Horsley have described it as having 'near hegemonic status among child and family practitioners'.[106] The UK government has claimed that a secure attachment (note the use of the singular again) 'contributes to good physical and mental health, speech and language development, emotional self-regulation, resilience and wider social and economic advantages throughout the life course'.[107] At the time of writing, health authorities in Scotland and Wales are committed to promoting secure attachments.[108] A key priority of the Healthy Child Wales Programme is 'to promote bonding and attachment to support positive parent-child relationships resulting in secure emotional attachment for children'.[109]

But, as we have seen, the 'truths' of attachment theory are anything but. Key assumptions remain unproven – and may even be unprovable. Although attachment promoters confidently assert that sensitive parenting builds attachment, the evidence simply doesn't back this up. It is dogma wrapped in a scientific mantle. The internal working model is undeveloped and needs to be treated as a working hypothesis, rather than a magical device which explains how mothers screw their children up. Insecure attachments do not inevitably lead to poor outcomes. Secure early attachments do not offer magical protection to children.

These issues are reflected in the confusing and inconsistent way in which attachment is measured and reported. Some researchers use three attachment categories, others four. Some collapse all the insecure categories into one to enable comparisons between secure and insecure.[110] The attachment categories are given different names by different researchers; for instance, 'avoidant' is variously known as 'anxious-avoidant', 'defended' or 'dismissing'. A systematic review of interventions for severe attachment problems observes that it is not always clear whether authors are creating new categories with subtle differences or simply renaming existing categories. This makes the literature on attachment 'extremely confusing'.

The review found a 'very large number' of different instruments used to classify attachments. Even Ainsworth's Strange Situation procedure has been subject to 'numerous' redesigns; the review counted twelve different versions of it in sixteen studies.[111] As we have already seen, other researchers have identified fifty different ways to measure sensitivity in early childhood.

Despite all its shortcomings, attachment theory has provided a rich framework to consider how babies, children and adults relate to each other. At the heart of it is Bowlby's observation that 'the propensity to make intimate emotional bonds to particular individuals [is] a basic component of human nature'.[112]

I wonder how much attachment theory shaped how I was mothered as a child. My mum was very affectionate with me and my brother, both physically and verbally (we were cuddled a lot and she used to say, 'I love you to pieces', which as a literal-minded child I found a little puzzling). She owned the 1965 edition of Bowlby's *Child Care and the Growth of Love* (which I now have), and Bowlby and Ainsworth influenced her work as a health visitor. One of her favourite phrases was 'it's impossible to spoil a baby', and she firmly believed that responding to babies' cries made them more secure and less clingy (a belief which I think can be traced back to a 1972 Ainsworth paper).[113] I wish she was still here so I could ask her how much attachment thinking actively influenced her mothering, or whether it simply validated what she would have done anyway.

We need relationships. But attachment theory cannot and should not be used to tell mothers how to interact with their babies. As Heidi Keller argues, attachment theory needs to shift from the view that attachment is a universal human need that operates in the same way everywhere to regarding it as a universal human need that looks and works differently across different cultures.[114] A secure base and safe haven can be provided in many different ways.

From both a policy and a research perspective, supporting relationships is not about micromanaging the interactions between parents and their children, but instead looking at what the academics Vivian Carlson and Robin Harwood call the 'systems of support' that enable or inhibit caregivers from successfully protecting and socialising their children.

For individual mothers, it's about making children feel cared for and safe – in whatever way they think is best. As Carlson and Harwood put it, 'Secure attachment relationships . . . develop in the context of trust and confidence on the part of the infant that the caregiver will provide comfort and protection when needed.'[115] It's as simple as that.

What stops it from being simple is all the things that get in the way; hunger, violence, addiction, poor housing, poverty, mental health problems and dangerous neighbourhoods can all be barriers to giving children comfort and protection. The solution is not sensitivity training but improving the fabric of people's lives.

The relationship between parents and children should only be someone else's business in cases of abuse or neglect, or where parents themselves ask for help because of, for instance, their own traumatic childhoods or they are concerned about their child. And here, as the academics Sue White, Matthew Gibson, David Wastell and Patricia Walsh argue, the use of attachment theory in child welfare practice needs to steer clear of pathologising 'diverse ranges of behaviour'. It should instead be put into a wider context 'respecting familial relational networks, seeking to develop, strengthen and deepen those relationships that provide connection and belonging'.[116]

Babies and children deserve to be loved and cared for. That's a moral imperative, not a scientific one. And their parents and other caregivers need an environment – a safe and nurturing garden to use a metaphor we will explore in the next chapter – to be able to provide that comfort, protection and support.

6

Babies Don't Need to Be Built

What role do parents have in their babies' development? The answer to that very much depends on who you ask. In a qualitative study of mothers of two-month-old babies from five different countries, Sara Harkness and Charles Super observed that baby development was viewed 'through distinctively different cultural lenses'.

For American and Korean mothers, the focus was on brain development. The American mothers typically stimulated their babies through providing plenty of interesting objects, in accordance with expert advice. Korean mothers saw themselves as direct sources of stimulation, for instance showing things to their babies or playing music to them. For Italian and Spanish mothers, development was more about nurturing social qualities. Spanish mothers talked of taking their babies 'to the street' to vary the baby's environment and to give them sensory, visual and auditory stimulation in a social setting. Dutch mothers, in contrast, emphasised the importance of healthy development through a calm environment and regular rest. If pictures were shown to babies, this was intended to calm not stimulate them.[1]

Current Western orthodoxies about child development – and Good Mother myths about what children need – disregard the huge variation in child-rearing practices across cultures and over the ages. Universal assumptions are common. For example, a study exploring the neurobiological basis of human attachment refers to 'species-typical maternal behaviours', such as gazing at the baby's face and 'motherese'-style, high-pitched vocalisations.[2] But the assertion that this behaviour is 'species-typical' is contradicted by the ethnographic record. In some cultures, mothers do not spend time gazing at their babies or talking to them. The academic Heidi Keller, who has researched child development in many cultures, describes a very different set of maternal behaviours to Western norms: 'Childcare [is] a co-occurring activity with extensive body contact and body stimulation, little face-to-face interaction, little verbal monitoring, and little object stimulation. The child is never alone, but also never the centre of attention.'[3]

The sociologist André Turmel has described psychology as 'an ahistorical and acultural domain grounded in the assumption of a universal child'.[4] Prevailing theories of child development are stripped of culture and context, obscuring the moral directives that underpin them and the circumstances that constrain parents. Factors such as poverty, racism and ill health are simply ignored.

The Modern Prescription to Play

Play is a particularly glaring example of our blinkered views about child development. It is unhesitatingly regarded as essential for development. There was near universal agreement that play is important for development and that parents should make time to play with their babies in research conducted by the NCT among UK parents when their babies were eight months and twenty-one months old (declaration of interest – I was on the steering group for this research project). Around 99% of mothers and fathers concurred with these two statements at both time points the research was carried out. Only around 40% thought that play should just be for fun.[5]

Cultural prescriptions on play are strong. A good example of this is Margot Sunderland's book *What Every Parent Needs to*

Know. Sunderland, who is a child psychologist and psycho-therapist, claims that parents need to 'activate' the 'PLAY system' and 'SEEKING system' in their child's brain. The warnings of not doing so are stark: 'Too many children grow up leading ordinary lives, but not ... the extraordinary ones that they may be capable of.'[6]

However, there is a lack of strong evidence demonstrating the benefits of play. 'The jury is still out' is the verdict of the authors of the academic textbook of developmental psychology, *Understanding Child Development*. Their judgement is that the evidence for strong cognitive benefits is not convincing, although it is more so for social competence. They conclude that whatever the developmental consequences of play might be, it is enjoyable for participants and observers, and this is its enduring value.[7] But play is not valued because it is pleasurable. Alison Gopnik notes a puritan streak in America where simple pleasures are turned into 'strenuous work projects'; middle-class parents only allow themselves to play if it is part of the work of parenting.[8]

Advice on play can be very prescriptive, Sunderland's particularly so. She says that children should not be left to get on with playing by themselves or with other children. She makes the bizarre claim that physical play with an adult is better than with a child because 'your adult responses, with your more advanced frontal lobe functions, will be more attuning than those of a child'. If a child is engaged in play, parents should not walk past but must comment. However, they should not ask questions in case they interrupt the child's flow. Choosing toys for a child and leading play are 'very common mistakes' as this apparently activates stress hormones for the child.

Sunderland appears to be blissfully unaware both of the strong drive in children to play and the absence of parent–child play in many cultures. The historical and anthropological record shows that parents do not play with their babies in most societies and parent-toddler play is, as the anthropologist David Lancy puts it, 'virtually non-existent'. Indeed, the !Kung people, upheld by some as exemplars of 'natural parenting', believe that playing with children is potentially harmful to their development. Play is often regarded as a 'welcome distraction' which keeps children out of the way so parents can get on with their work. Lancy describes the notion that children need to be 'taught' how to play as 'absurd' and 'ridiculous'. Conflict-ridden societies are a rare exception to parents involving themselves in children's play; in these societies violent play is encouraged to socialise children to become aggressive.[9]

In Western culture, it was only in modern times that play activities came to be seen as the preserve of children. Historically play was, in the words of the historian Gary Cross, 'a periodic catharsis, associated with fairs and festivals rather than with childhood'. He observes how industrialisation led to specialised workplaces, creating a greater delineation between work and leisure. Children, especially from the emerging middle classes, withdrew from the labour market to attend school and began to enjoy opportunities for holidays and play.[10]

While play became associated with children, it took longer for this to become the responsibility of parents. Indeed, playing with babies was once actively discouraged. 'Do not encourage your baby to play before the second year' was the advice in a pamphlet called *Hints to Mothers Who Want Better Babies*, published in the 1910s by the US magazine *The Woman's Home Companion*.[11] The paediatrician Luther Emmett Holt's best-selling book *The Care and Feeding of Children* was first published in 1894 and went through twelve revisions by the mid-1920s.[12] He warned that babies under six months should never be played with because this would make them 'nervous and irritable, sleep badly and suffer from indigestion and in many other respects'. If young children were going to be played with at all, this should be in the morning or after the midday nap. He made brain claims of a very different hue to what we hear today. He argued that the 'delicate structure' of the brain and its rapid growth requires 'quiet and peaceful surroundings' in order to prevent 'excessive nervousness'.[13]

It was only in the post–Second World War era that expert advice turned play into a new duty for mothers, wittily described by the psychologist Martha Wolfenstein as the 'fun morality'.[14] The historian Peter Stearns partly attributes the growing obligation of parents to entertain their children to the rise of consumerism and the efforts of advertisers ('buy this, take them there, and you'll know from their joy that you're a really good parent'). Other factors were that children were less able to organise their own activities outside the home and smaller families meant fewer siblings to play with.[15]

'Fun morality' neatly encompasses the practical and emotional responsibilities mothers are supposed to assume around play. For some women, playing with their babies and children can be pleasurable and reassuring – as the psychotherapist Rozsika Parker puts it, 'a beacon of certainty in the sea of motherhood . . . a sense of being in possession of a reliable tool of the trade'.[16] But for others, as Parker observes, it is a source of guilt, anxiety and boredom. This guilt can be intensified by expert advice that ignores the possibility that children's play can be dull for adults. For instance, Sunderland informs us that playing is so rewarding for parents they will inevitably want to do it more: 'Once you have managed to activate the PLAY system in your child's brain, her squeals of delight will soon be so reinforcing that you will both want more playtimes like this.'[17]

Attention-seeking?

Parents, and particularly mothers, are expected to lavish babies and young children with attention. This is another culturally shaped belief, a Good Mother myth specific to the modern era. What is required from parents today was regarded as most inadvisable in Victorian times. Mothers and fathers were warned that 'the restless over-anxiety of parents to excite and amuse very young children' could cause 'nervous susceptibility . . . ultimately becoming the source of great distress of both mind and body'.

This is from *The Management of Infancy: Physiological and Moral,* the popular Victorian work we met in previous chapters. It highlights the dangers in making a child 'unceasingly the object of the exclusive attention of those around it': 'Its self-esteem, thus early and assiduously fostered, becomes daily more dominant and exacting; and, in proportion as the infant feels its power, it becomes a tyrant in its own petty sphere.'[18]

Concerns about the potential physical and emotional harm of over-stimulation echoed down the years. Sydney Frankenburg, the expert we encountered in the first chapter, equated this to cruelty, warning of perils, such as 'badly-built teeth':

> Over-stimulation, next to deliberate cruelty and persistent neglect, is the most harmful treatment to which a child can be subjected . . . Among the more serious physical effects of over-stimulation are badly-built teeth, the result of diverting to the brain the blood that should have been used for body-building.[19]

Frankenburg instead recommended some 'wholesome neglect'. By 1946, when she wrote the final edition of her manual, wholesome neglect was falling out of fashion. The developmental paradigm was changing. In the words of historian Stephen Lassonde, faith in children's 'innate resilience' was being displaced by the belief that children are 'fragile and requiring constant attention'.[20]

This shift had its roots in economic changes and the withdrawal of middle-class children from the labour market. In the sociologist Viviana Zelizer's memorable and often-quoted observation, 'the twentieth-century economically useless but emotionally priceless child displaced the nineteenth-century useful child.'[21] The historian Julia Grant puts it another way – the dynamic changed from children serving their parents to parents serving their children.[22]

To return to my earlier metaphor of the tightrope, parents were required to be attentive but not excessively so because concerns about giving children too much attention endured. In all seven editions of his manual published during his lifetime (from 1946 to 1998), Dr Spock warned against 'a steady flow of fussy attention' because this can spoil children in two ways:

> He grows up assuming that he is the hub of the universe and that everyone should automatically admire him whether he is being attractive or not. On the other hand, he hasn't been practising how to make his own fun or how to be outgoing and appealing to people.[23]

From the second edition onwards, Spock included a section on what he called 'unspoiling'. He advised mothers to busy themselves for most of the time the baby is awake ('with housework or anything else'). If the baby frets or wants to be carried, the mother should say in a 'friendly but very firm tone' that she has jobs to do. Spock concedes that this may be difficult:

> It takes a lot of willpower and a little hardening of the heart. To get yourself in the right mood you have to remember that, in the long run, unreasonable demandingness and excessive dependence are worse for babies than for you. They make him out of sorts with himself and the world.[24]

Spock was criticised for being too child-centred and permissive on discipline, charges which were in part politically inspired because of his anti-war and civil rights activism. These accusations were a cause of great frustration to him, both professionally and personally (he told an interviewer 'I was a stern, stern father').[25] It is a sign of how much attitudes have changed that the political attacks against Spock in the 1960s for producing a permissive 'Spock-marked generation' could have any currency at all. Now, Spock would be criticised for advocating childcare practices which fail to 'optimise' infant brains.

Why the Brain Is Not a House

Parents nowadays are expected to build their babies – and their brains. Building metaphors pervade advice about babies. For instance, UNICEF UK (whose brain claims we have already encountered in Chapter 1) has published a leaflet called *Building a Happy Baby*. This states that the responsibility to build brains begins before a baby has even been born: 'You can help your baby's brain development during pregnancy by talking, reading, stroking and playing music.'[26]

'Remember, you're building her mind,' an instructor tells Frida, the protagonist of Jessamine Chan's novel *The School for Good Mothers*. Frida has been sent to a facility for mothers and has been issued with a robotic child on which to practise her parenting skills. Her instructors school her on strengthening her child-first orientation and stimulating her doll's curiosity with developmentally appropriate, loving and insightful questions. The doll collects data on Frida, who is warned any negative feelings will impede her progress and that she must also relax because her heart rate shows she is stressed. Frida was sentenced to a year in the facility because she left her eighteen-month-old daughter alone for a couple of hours. The judge admonished her that her daughter's brain may develop differently because of this.[27] Chan's book brilliantly satirises how cruel and absurd Good Mother myths can be.

The building metaphor was dreamed up by the communication-savvy groups we encountered in Chapter 2, the Harvard Center on the Developing Child and its related body the National Scientific Council on the Developing Child. It underpins a narrative which lays at the feet of parents the job of building, moulding and sculpting their children's brains. The starting point is 'brain architecture', as a 2007 paper sets out: 'The quality of a child's early environment and the availability of appropriate experiences at the right stages of development are crucial in determining the strength or weakness of the brain's architecture.' The concept of a house is then deployed to explain the perils of defective brain wiring: 'Just as a faulty foundation has far-reaching detrimental effects on the strength and quality of a house, adverse early experience can have far-reaching detrimental effects on the development of brain architecture.'[28]

The edict to ensure children's brains are wired properly is used to justify all sorts of prescriptions, notably the micromanagement of interactions between parents and children. This is through the concept of 'serve and return', which is another of the simplifying models developed by FrameWorks and the Harvard Center on the Developing Child.

Serve and return happens 'when young children naturally reach out for interaction through babbling, facial expressions, words, gestures, and cries, and adults respond by getting in sync and doing the same kind of vocalizing and gesturing back at them, and the process continues back and forth.'[29] It is claimed that these interactions are 'fundamental to the wiring of the brain'.[30]

But 'serve and return' does not accord with the ethnographic record, as we have seen. It also makes little evolutionary sense – if parents had spent their time ensuring they smiled and babbled every time their baby smiled and babbled, we would not have got very far. And there is no consideration for the different ways babies and adults relate to each other or space for questions or doubts. As a parent, how well am I equipping my children for the world if I 'return' every time they 'serve'? Recall Dr Spock's concerns about children growing up assuming they are 'the hub of the universe'. More practically, how are parents supposed to deal with the many other demands on their time and energy if they are constantly serving and returning? The time of parents, particularly mothers, is assumed to be a boundless resource.

Concepts such as 'brain architecture' and 'serve and return' are shielded from criticism and scrutiny because they are presented as scientific fact. But neuroscience is in its infancy, the science is far from settled and there is much we have yet to learn about the human brain. What we *can* say is that the brain is anything but a house built from the bottom up. It is a plastic living organism which changes throughout life. Time-lapse studies on the brain in animals show that, in the words of Hilary and Steven Rose, synapses are 'highly dynamic, continually being modified, disappearing and being reformed throughout life . . . This remodelling capacity – plasticity – is the neural mechanism that enables a person to learn from experience, remember and change how they respond.'[31]

Matthew Cobb points out the limits of metaphors of the brain as a computer or a machine:

> Brains, unlike any machine, have not been designed. They are organs that have evolved for over five hundred million years, so there is little or no reason to expect they truly function like the machines we create . . . The scale of complexity of even the simplest of brains dwarfs any machine we can currently envisage.

A house is a particularly clunky and inadequate metaphor for something as complex and mysterious as the brain. As we saw in an earlier chapter, we still don't really know how simple nervous systems like the gastric mill in a lobster's stomach work. This demonstrates how far we have to go in understanding how the human brain develops. Cobb says, 'Given our poor understanding of even very simple nervous systems, unravelling the genetic architecture of the human brain and how it interacts with the environment will be the work of centuries.'[32] There is a yawning gap between the state of our actual knowledge of the brain and the confident certainty with which the decrees about building babies' brains are made. The strength of the metaphor is cultural, not scientific. It derives its power and credibility from Good Mother myths, not scientific knowledge. The belief that women can sculpt their children's brains appeals to our desire for neat explanations and simple solutions.

The house metaphor is a new iteration of 'tabula rasa', the baby as a blank slate. It ignores genetic influences and the role of chance in how individual brains develop. The neurogeneticist Kevin Mitchell explains how individual variation in how neural systems develop is down to both genetic differences in the programme specifying brain development and function, and random variation in how that program plays out in an individual: 'In short, we're born different from each other.'

Mitchell makes it clear that this is not about genetic determinism. Rather, there are differences in what he calls 'innate behavioural predispositions' which are shaped by experiences and environment. Parents cannot mould their children's personalities, but they can 'certainly influence the way they adapt to the world'. Mitchell ends his book *Innate: How the Wiring of Our Brains Shapes Who We Are* with a plea to accept ourselves and each other:

> We're shy, smart, wild, kind, anxious, impulsive, hardworking, absent-minded, quick-tempered. We literally see the world differently, think differently, and feel things differently. Some of us make our way through the world with ease, and some of us struggle to fit in or get along or keep it together. Denying those differences or constantly telling people they should change is not helpful to anyone. We should recognize the diversity of our human natures, accept it, embrace it, even celebrate it.[33]

Science-based Brain Building Tips or Science-induced Guilt Trips?

The brain claims developed by the Harvard Center on the Developing Child support a thriving early intervention industry which instructs parents on how to interact with their children. Vroom, a global programme funded by the Bezos Family Foundation, 'provides science-based tips and tools to inspire families to turn shared, everyday moments into Brain Building Moments®'.[34]

The NSPCC has adopted the Vroom approach wholesale for its Look, Say, Sing, Play campaign which tells parents, 'You've got the power to change everyday moments into brain-building ones.' But this is nonsense – the everyday moments the NSPCC talks about, such as bath time or going to the shops, *do* stimulate children, regardless of whether parents are consciously trying to make them into 'brain-building' experiences.[35]

What all these programmes, campaigns and 'tips' boil down to is an admonition to 'do more' and to do so consciously with the aim of 'optimising' development. As we have seen, the concept of 'optimising' runs through current orthodoxy about child development, with 'the more the better' exhorted implicitly or explicitly. For instance, the NSPCC tells us, 'Right from birth, every time you talk, sing or play with your baby, you're not just bonding, you're building their brain.'[36] The implication is that every time you don't do these things, your baby's brain is not being built.

The Good Mother myth that the more stimulation a baby receives the better is a logical fallacy. There is a ceiling to how far anything can develop or grow, it cannot be infinite. If this myth goes unchallenged, it means that whatever parents – particularly mothers – do, it is never enough. We will always be found wanting.

Margot Sunderland's book *What Every Parent Needs to Know*, which we met earlier in the chapter, is an excellent example of the pressures that the brain optimisation narrative puts on mothers, as well as the prescriptive nonsense that is rammed down people's throats.[37]

The evangelical title of the book says it all (the US edition is called *The Science of Parenting: How Today's Brain Research Can Help You Raise Happy, Emotionally Balanced Children*). Sunderland says she wants to 'empower parents to make informed choices'. But really, she just wants to tell parents what to do; 'informed choices' actually means providing 'evidence' to ensure that parents make what Sunderland regards as the correct choices. She writes, 'It's too easy to choose some commonly accepted child-rearing practices, which can damage a child's brain and body. This book is here to help ensure you don't do that!'

Sunderland then goes on to hit the reader over the head with neuroscience and guilt-inducing claims. We are told that it is up to parents whether their children's brains are wired for calm or alarm. In a section entitled 'Parenting the Brain', Sunderland writes: 'Your approach can determine whether or not your child's brain systems and brain chemistries are activated in such a way as to enable him to enjoy a rich and rewarding life.'

The book is a flurry of brain diagrams and footnotes to research studies. This gives it the veneer of scientific credibility (I have heard it praised for having 'masses of science'). However, Sunderland makes claims that are not backed up in any way at all by the studies she cites. For instance, we are told, 'The more responsive you are, the greater your regulation of her body arousal systems will be, and the more long-lasting the effects.' Two studies are cited in support of this statement. One relates to the timing of skin-to-skin contact at birth so tells us nothing about long-term effects.[38] The other is a study investigating the link between maternal sensitivity during the first three years of life and social and academic competence at the age of thirty-two.[39] It has nothing to do with body arousal systems or any other element of physiology. There is absolutely nothing to back up Sunderland's contention of 'the more the better', which in any case fails on the grounds of logic alone.

Sunderland's extravagant assertions about the benefits of co-sleeping are another example. Children who have co-slept with their parents apparently have higher self-esteem, experience less fear and anxiety, perform better cognitively, suffer from fewer mental health issues in adulthood and enjoy a greater feeling of satisfaction with life. These are quite some claims, but of the three studies cited in support, two are rodent studies and the other looks at bed-sharing and non-bed-sharing between two and twenty-four weeks after birth.[40]

There are always rat studies as I quickly came to learn when I started looking under the bonnet of neuroscience narratives. Sunderland, like other pedlars of brain claims, relies heavily on animal research and often fails to acknowledge this. For instance, she tells us, 'Research shows that if a child's need for comfort is not met with emotional responsiveness and soothing, this system can, over time, become wired for bodily hyperarousal.' The study cited in support of this claim summarises research among rats and primates, not children.[41] I will say it once again – we women are not chimpanzees, and our children are not rats.

Sunderland's repeated references to particular parts of the brain to frame her arguments is another common tactic in the brain claims industry. The neuroscientist Paul Fletcher has described this as 'neuro-flapdoodle', in which 'a highly simplistic and questionable point is accompanied by a suitably grand-sounding neural term and thus acquires a weightiness that it really doesn't deserve'.[42] As the academics David Wastell and Sue White point out, multiple brain regions are generally involved in any given psychological process, ruling out simplistic relation-ships such as that of the amygdala with violence.[43]

Sunderland uses the cloak of science to moralise and set enor-mously high standards. Parents should '*always* [my emphasis] be thinking about how you come over to your child'. They are urged to monitor how many 'high-intensity positive relational moments' they are having with their child with a handy assessment tool provided by Sunderland. There is no recognition of other pulls on time such as other children or work, or the constraints parents face because of factors such as poverty, racism, ill health and disability.

Like many experts, Sunderland's advice floats in a vacuum, free of the gravity of context or culture. She assumes that parents have endless time and resources. If a child is making a magic potion with flour and water on the kitchen floor, their parent shouldn't tell them to tidy up but should support them by giving them props, such as jugs and more rice or cereal to add to their potion. There is no consideration of the possibility that it may be the last bag of flour and there's no money left until payday or that the parent has other things to do. As the sociologist Tracey Jensen points out, parenting advice ignores the socioeconomic realities of people's lives.[44]

There is a real lack of compassion in some of what Sunderland says. For instance, she claims that the reason why some parents don't fall in love with their new baby as soon as it is born is 'often because they don't believe a baby is all that interesting until she begins to talk'. There is no recognition that it is normal to feel detached after birth, particularly after an exhausting or traumatic labour.[45]

Similarly, Sunderland does not acknowledge that looking after small children can be boring – if you are longing for peace, it is because you are biochemically 'dysregulated'. Sunderland suggests that vitamins may be the answer: 'When you find yourself over-reacting to your child's behaviour, ask yourself, "is my child annoying me because of a stressful situation, or am I short of some key vitamins?"' If only vitamins were the answer to the many difficulties mothers face.

Although it is easy enough to poke fun at Sunderland's book, her arguments are taken deadly seriously. Like Sue Gerhardt's *Why Love Matters*, which we looked at in a previous chapter, it features on reading lists for health visitors and midwives.[46] Both these books contribute to a culture where women are always found wanting and their efforts discounted. As Jan Macvarish says, 'The demands on women's time, labour and emotions by the need for constant love and nurture are rendered even less negotiable by the threat of long-term, biologically rooted damage to their children's brains.'[47] The supposed danger of damaged brains fuels Good Mother myths of boundless sacrifice and supplies fertile territory for mother blame.

Saving Brains by Building 'Appropriate Neural Pathways'

Although neuroscience is presented as cutting edge, it is fuelled by a sense of evangelism with deep historical roots. The academics Val Gillies, Rosalind Edwards and Nicola Horsley see clear echoes of Victorian moral crusades to rescue children from their 'irredeemable parents', although the 'tussles are now over brains rather than souls'.[48]

Badly wired brains instead of inferior stock now preoccupy politicians. As we saw in Chapter 2, brain claims came to life as a political project in the US in the 1990s and have captivated politicians and policymakers ever since. The title of the 2015 report *Building Great Britons: Conception to the Age of 2* is redolent of the concerns a century ago about the fitness of the British population. The report was published by the First 1001 Days All-Party Parliamentary Group with support from politicians of all parties. It asserts that 'decisive action be taken to ensure the proportion of good citizens rises sharply in the future'. Building better brains is what is required:

> Parents who are able to understand their baby's cues and tune into their baby's needs are able to provide the responses and experiences that their baby needs at different points in their baby's life in order to support the establishment of appropriate neural pathways and optimal development of their baby's brain.[49]

The implication is that parents who do not tune into their baby's needs will end up with children whose brains are suboptimal and have 'inappropriate' neural pathways. Bad citizens have bad brains. As we saw in Chapter 1, health professionals used to preach strict feeding schedules to breed good character, but now the emphasis is on constant, attentive mothering to produce well-adjusted citizens. In their qualitative research among early years practitioners, Gillies, Edwards and Horsley found a sincere commitment to the potential of 'brain science' to transform the lives of parents and children: 'A fervent enthusiasm and belief in vocation characterised their descriptions of their work that could echo the language of evangelism and biology.'[50]

Brain claims are used to justify removing babies and young children from their apparently irredeemable families. As we saw in Chapter 1, the number of newborn babies removed from their mothers in England has shot up, and one factor behind this is a research review commissioned by the Department of Education and the Family Justice Council for professionals involved in care orders. Although the review admits that knowledge about how parenting influences brain development is still embryonic, it presents the evidence in confident terms, drawing heavily on the work of the Harvard Center on the Developing Child and citing Sue Gerhardt:

> Environment and experiences have the greatest impact during the first three years of a child's life, particularly during the first year, when the brain is developing most rapidly . . . because very young children are so dependent on adults for survival, the attachment formed with the primary caregiver (usually the mother) shapes the way in which the brain develops.[51]

Critiques of the review by academics such as David Wastell and Sue White were rebuffed for undermining the case for more timely intervention to protect children.[52] We must not leave it too late to save their brains.

Evangelical 'brain science' has also fuelled the export of Western parenting norms to other parts of the world. We came across the 'Nurturing Care Framework' in the previous chapter. This was adopted in 2018 by the World Health Organization, UNICEF and the World Bank Group. The framework, we are told, 'draws on state-of-the-art evidence on how early childhood development unfolds'. It is intended to be used as a 'roadmap for action'. Investing in early childhood (defined as the first three years) is, apparently, 'one of the most efficient and effective ways to help eliminate extreme poverty and inequality'.

'Responsive caregiving' – 'observing and responding to children's movements, sounds and gestures and verbal requests' – is a core component of the Nurturing Care Framework. It is claimed that this type of caregiving is 'essential for the optimal [that word again] development of the baby's rapidly growing brain'.[53] This illustrates how Good Mother myths fashioned from attachment theory are then buttressed by brain claims.

These arguments are used to justify international development programmes in the Global South which target parents, and particularly mothers.[54] For example, Saving Brains (note the crusading name), a philanthropic organisation funded by the Bill and Melinda Gates Foundation among others, has sponsored a programme in Nigeria entitled *Family-Inclusive Early Brain Stimulation* (giving us the snappy acronym 'FInE BrainS'). Its aim is to teach parents to interact with their children 'better':

> Social interactions in the form of 'serve and return' exchanges between child and parent serve as building blocks for psychosocial, physical and cognitive development. Parents in sub-Saharan countries are ill-equipped to maximise the benefits from this interaction.

This is astonishingly patronising and demeaning, failing to understand how – let alone why – children from non-Western cultures are cared for in different ways from Western cultural norms. As Gillies, Edwards and Horsley point out, it 'smacks of imperialism'.[55] This intrusion into the relationships between women and their children is justified on the grounds that 'early life experiences drive the development of brain architecture' and 'poor stimulation and poor social interaction can affect brain structure and function, and have lasting cognitive and emotional effects.'[56] The evidence cited in support is, predictably, a 2007 paper by the National Scientific Council on the Developing Child (which we came across in Chapter 2) and, of course, a rat study.[57]

What Babies Really Need

A great fraud is being perpetrated on parents, and particularly women, because ordinary, loving care is all typically developing babies need. As the academics Alison Gopnik, Andrew Meltzoff and Patricia Kuhl argue in *The Scientist in the Crib*: 'Our instinctive behaviours toward babies and babies' instinctive behaviours toward us combine to enable the babies to learn as much as they do.'[58] The developmental psychologist Lynne Murray makes a similar point – much of what we do when we engage with babies is outside our conscious awareness but is often 'very complex and tuned to the baby's abilities in a way that precisely supports their development'.[59]

Building metaphors also obscure children's drive to learn and their ability to absorb what they need to develop. To quote from *The Scientist in the Crib* again: 'Babies are already as smart as they can be, they know what they need to know and they are very effective and selective in getting the kinds of information they need.' Children have 'a kind of explanatory drive . . . [which] pushes them to act in ways that will get them the information they need; it leads them to explore and experiment'.

One of my favourite examples of this is something called body babbling, where babies carefully watch their body movements to help them figure out the relationship between the feeling of moving a particular part of their body and what it looks like. For instance, at around two to three months of age, babies can be fascinated by observing their hands moving.[60]

Another glorious example is the remarkable ability of typically developing babies to learn language. Steven Pinker argues that 'language acquisition is a stubbornly robust process; from what we can tell there is virtually no way to prevent it from happening short of raising a child in a barrel'.[61] Babies are sponges, with an amazing capacity to absorb how language works. This begins in the womb, with one study finding that the cries of newborn babies from French- and German-speaking families sound different. The study analysed the cries of sixty babies at two to five days of age, with half recruited from French-speaking families and half from German-speaking families. The French babies' cries had a rising melody contour, whereas the German group produced falling contours.[62] Language acquisition proceeds rapidly; babies as young as six months are able to recognise simple words such as apple.[63]

Adults intuitively support this process through parentese/motherese (also known as 'infant-directed speech'). Adults unconsciously speak in a particular way when they are talking to babies – in short sentences, with repetition, using a sing-song higher pitch and exaggerated, lengthened vowels. This is thought to help children grasp the words and grammar of their language and is universal in all cultures where adults speak to children (not all do).[64] It is a great example of what caregivers do to support their babies' development without realising it.

I wish I had known more about the amazing abilities of babies when my children were little. More awe and less anxiety would have made my experience of early motherhood so much more enjoyable. For instance, from about two months babies understand that objects are solid and are already sensitive to numbers of items.[65] I also wish I had appreciated how I, and the other loving adults in my children's lives, were supporting their development, as well as how much of their development was down to them. Learning about baby development is, as Lynne Murray argues, intrinsically fascinating, but it also affirms the 'immense value of what parents do, day in day out'.

There is very little research about the feelings of women on brain claims or on development more broadly – which is telling. A key learning from an evaluation of the *Five to Thrive* programme at two Barnardo's family centres is that the parents thought that instructions on how to build their children's brains were not particularly helpful. The programme teaches parents that there are five 'building blocks' for a healthy brain: Respond, Cuddle, Relax, Play, Talk. These are, of course, things that parents are doing anyway. So it is perhaps not very surprising that the evaluation concluded that 'many parents felt that they learnt more from meeting with other parents to discuss the "realities" of parenting'.[66]

Other research highlights that mothers can feel anxious about not doing enough to help their children's development. The sociologist Glenda Wall's qualitative research among Canadian mothers of pre-schoolers found that most mothers accepted without question a sense of responsibility for their children's outcomes. Many worried that if they did not do everything they could to stimulate their children's development, this would hamper their future prospects.[67]

There is an interesting nugget in qualitative research that Steph Lawler did in the 1990s among British mothers which suggests that mothers can disregard what they do to support their babies' development. Women felt that practical tasks such as nappy changing hardly counted as 'mothering' at all. It was emotional care which they saw as most important.[68] But nappy changing stimulates a baby's senses and helps them map together the different parts of their body. It is an example of one of the many ways in which parents help their children's development without realising it.

Nevertheless, if day-to-day activities like nappy changing are not intentionally done to stimulate development, they can be discounted. In one of my postnatal groups, I remember a woman saying she was really worried that she was not spending enough time stimulating her baby. As she talked, she gently played with her baby's hand, stroking each finger in turn. When I mentioned this, she said it had not occurred to her that this simple, unconscious, loving interaction supported her baby's development.

My experience of running postnatal groups among new mothers is that baby development provokes strong feelings of anxiety and inadequacy. What should I be doing, and when, and how much, and what should I buy? Baby classes, which are heavily marketed to mothers as having developmental benefits, are one way to try to counter the pressure. Andrea O'Reilly argues that by filling up their days with activities like Gymboree classes, women are doing things that 'can be documented as productive and visible work'.[69]

As well as piling on the guilt and pressure, telling parents to build their babies can suck the fun out of life. As Charlotte Faircloth says:

> Providing children with the right kind of environment turns normal activities of parenting into a series of tasks to be achieved. Touching, talking and feeding are no longer ends in themselves, but tools mothers are required to perfect to ensure optimal development.[70]

The focus on sculpting and building babies with an eye to the future gets in the way of the here and now – the great joy there is to be had in the moment with children. The Good Mother myth that babies need to be built undermines the pleasurable experiences of mothering.

The building narrative also offers very little to parents of children who are not developing typically or who have chronic illnesses. A qualitative Australian study among mothers of twins and triplets with special needs found, 'With the early years normally being a time of rapid development, the opportunities for fresh heartbreak were many.'[71] André Turmel notes that developmental milestones such as walking and talking are based on the assumption of the typically developing 'normal' child, with normal conveying the meanings of healthy and acceptable, as well as average.

Like the word natural, the word 'normal' carries with it a cruelty if it is absent – if you are not normal, you are abnormal. The sociologist Angela Frederick uses the term 'normalcy project' to describe a regime of beliefs and practices 'which are preoccupied with eradicating disability and which prize a typical body'.[72] Both she and Turmel note the use of the language of statistics in child development – averages, norms and deviations from the norm.[73]

The milestones may be different and later, but the development of disabled or chronically ill children is no less precious or important to their families and should be valued and celebrated. Life can be a whirl of hospital appointments and struggles to access the right services, equipment and treatment. These children – and their parents – deserve to have what is needed to support their health, development and wellbeing.

We Need to Be Gardening Not Building

Babies do not need to be built, they need to be given the right conditions to grow and flourish. This is the central idea in Alison Gopnik's book *The Gardener and the Carpenter*. Gopnik argues that adults are gardeners rather than carpenters when it comes to bringing up children. The job of a gardener is to provide a protected and nurturing space for plants to flourish, and the same is required for children. They need a safe and stable environment to thrive. Gopnik maintains that we don't have to teach young children so much as to let them learn.[74]

Gopnik's metaphor works because it helps us think about all the things that can get in the way of mothers and fathers providing a nurturing garden, such as poverty, racism, abuse, ill health, poor housing and unsafe neighbourhoods. It shifts our focus to what parents need to enable them to support their children. This focus must be at both an individual and societal level. For instance, parents whose children are ill or not developing typically should not have to fight for the right support or therapy.

The belief that babies – and their brains – need to be built obscures all the factors which constrain children's life chances and puts women, in particular, under immense pressure. Brain claims have so much currency because they provide people who care passionately about children's futures seemingly simple ways to make things better. There is a more cynical side to this too;

making mothers responsible for building their children's brains is a convenient alibi for societal ills. But the emphasis on the intricacies of interactions between parents and children is a red herring, a Good Mother myth that we must reject. Our focus should be much more ambitious if we want to give all children the opportunity to blossom and bloom.

Conclusion

Embracing Motherdom

An End to Good Mother Myths

It took me a long time to work out that it is impossible to be a 'Good Mother'. Women are socialised to look inwardly for explanations if we think we are falling short. And Good Mother myths are so deeply embedded; they are an indiscernible part of our cultural and emotional landscape. In her book *Matrescence*, the writer Lucy Jones describes her realisation during pregnancy that 'something else had been accreting within me, too: a strange admixture of unexamined moral assumptions about motherhood . . . it became clear, once the baby was born, that I felt that self-sacrifice was an essential component of being a good mother'.[1]

The status of Good Mother is unattainable because the standards which mothers are held to are unrealistic and unforgiving. The yardsticks used to measure what is 'good' warp and shift according to who is being judged and who is doing the judging. Good Mother myths are endlessly mutable. An array of values and views on child-rearing means that women are always at risk of being told they are doing something wrong, whatever their actions. As the writer Deborah Levy observes of mothers: 'It is a miracle she survives our mixed messages, written in society's most poisoned ink. It is enough to drive her mad.'[2]

We need to destroy Good Mother myths. They are not just a problem for parents – the spectre of the Good Mother haunts all women. If we are to challenge the ideology of women as givers, we need to sweep away its underpinnings. Good Mother myths justify power structures where women are lesser, and caring work is both devalued and expected.

Enter Motherdom

Motherdom means setting mothers free. As Adrienne Rich said:

> To destroy the institution is not to abolish motherhood. It is to release the creation and sustenance of life into the same realm of decision, struggle, surprise, imagination, and conscious intelligence, as any other difficult, but freely chosen work.[3]

Motherdom offers a generous and expansive vision of motherhood. It is a concept of rich potential, which can carry a multiplicity of meanings. As I explained at the start of this book, notions of 'condition, state, dignity, domain and realm' are all contained within the word 'motherdom'.

Motherdom should be political as well as personal. The writer and self-described 'Queer Black Feminist Love Evangelist', Alexis Pauline Gumbs argues for 'the queerness of mothering as a practice itself' because it 'requires a person to change the status quo of their own lives, of their community and of the society as a whole again and again and again in the practice of affirming growing, unpredictable people who deserve a world that is better than what we can even imagine'.[4] This vision is exciting and inspiring, according mothers dignity and political power, and aspiring to a better future for our children.

In her review of the anthology Gumbs contributed to, Jennifer Nash says she is 'both seduced by and skeptical of the representation of black motherhood as radical and revolutionary, as spiritual and transformative'. Nash asks some incisive questions. How does revolutionary Black motherhood encompass a variety of maternal experiences including maternal ambivalence; how to avoid conflating Black mothers and Black women, thus neglecting women who are not mothers, and what place does maternal labour – 'uncompensated and oftentimes exhausting work' – have in all of this?[5] Nash raises important issues for us all. We must tread carefully in the domain of motherdom; Good Mother myths are hazardous landmines in the terrain we want to travel.

Motherhood is a reckoning – with the best and the worst of ourselves, with the society we live in now and the one we want our children to grow and prosper in. In the remainder of this chapter, I explore the concept of motherdom. It can be both a recognition of reality and an ideal. The many ways in which children and parents are failed by society need to be tackled. I end with a consideration of what our own personal motherdom can be.

Motherdom Is Glorious Variety and Diversity

Motherdom means recognising and valuing the many different ways in which mothers care for their children. What was written by the researchers Rhona and Robert N. Rapoport and Ziona Strelitz in 1977 in *Fathers, Mothers, and Others* (we discussed this book in Chapter 1) holds true today: 'People have different personality constellations, skills and interests. This implies that they are potentially capable of contributing to parental love and care in *various* ways while meeting both their children's and their own needs.'[6]

In order to dismantle Good Mother myths, we need to broaden and enrich our understanding of relationships between parents (not just mothers) and children. Parents nurture their children in so many different ways, such as through food, conversation, touch, reading and music. The writer Angela Garbes observes that 'love is an action verb . . . Mothering is acts of service and attention to the body. Drool wiping, hand washing, nose blowing, food spooning, hair brushing, bathing, picking up, pinning down to put clothes on, changing diapers.'[7]

There are also many ways in which mothers seek to protect their children, from ensuring they cross roads safely to schooling them in how to avoid police violence. In her essay 'Losing My

Mother Tongue: India and England', my friend Rupal Shah, a doctor and writer, says of her mother: 'Her way of expressing her love is not the same as mine; she shows her love through doing, I show my love for my daughters through words.' One of her mother's acts of love and protection was making Rupal packed lunches every day to take to her North London primary school. This was so she did not have to eat the strange English food that she was encountering for the first time: 'There was a grotesque purple pudding that made a lasting impression on me.'[8]

Motherdom also incorporates a variety of mothering identities and family set-ups. Andrea O'Reilly's theory of 'empowered mothering', includes 'a multitude of maternal identities, such as noncustodial, poor, single, young, old, and employed mothers, and a variety of motherhood practices, such as the practices of "othermothering" found in African American culture and the co-mothering of queer households'.[9]

Drawing inspiration from queer parenting can help dissolve maternal stereotypes and throw out biological essentialism (which underpins the myth of the natural). A child may have multiple parents. The writer Zena Sharman's child has four parents, none of whom identify as a mother. Each chose their parent moniker; Sharman's is ZeeZee, a variation on her first name. Sharman reflects: 'We found our way into a family structure that worked for all of us, an ongoing negotiation as we continue growing into our relationships with our child and with each other.'[10]

There are many, many ways to be a good mother. The scientist and writer Pragya Agarwal puts it beautifully: 'I want to feel and believe that I can design my motherhood the way I want to. My motherhood does not have to prove anything to anyone.'[11]

Motherdom means rejecting – fiercely – the idea that there is an 'optimal' way to care for babies and children. There isn't. There really isn't. Philosophically, politically and scientifically, optimisation makes no sense. Variation and diversity are at the heart of what it is to be human, and we see this in the many different ways women mother across and within different societies.

Without this rich variability, humans would not have been able to survive and thrive in so many different contexts.

Motherdom Is about Appreciating Everything Mothers Do for Their Children

Outside the realm of motherdom, mothers invariably fall short. This is deeply unfair. We need to switch from a deficit to a credit model, where the many things that women do for their children are acknowledged and appreciated. Women mothering in difficult circumstances deserve particular admiration for the determination and ingenuity they have to bring to bear (although admiration is no substitute for adequate support).

We need to ditch the dogma that we have to 'optimise' children's development by consciously doing things to stimulate them. Mary Ainsworth questioned this towards the end of her life: 'I don't think it's a very healthy thing to be *at* the child too much, to have him taste this and smell that and feel this, trying to enrich all aspects of his life . . . It's experience the child needs.'[12]

Babies and children are stimulated by whatever their mothers do for them and with them. Indeed, they are stimulated by *life*. In her history of childcare advice, the writer Christina Hardyment says there is a case for arguing that 'children thrive most as secure little spectators on adult lives rather than as the centre of anxious attention'.[13]

We focus – and Good Mother myths encourage us to have this focus – on the negatives, what we feel that we aren't getting right. Instead, we should appreciate all the love and care we give to our children. We should value the multitude of things we do for our children which benefits them in many different ways, which makes them feel cared for and safe.

We must also recognise the challenges which can make mothering so much harder; personal struggles such as ill health, bereavement or separation, as well as societal factors like poverty and racism. On an individual level, this means being compassionate to ourselves about our difficulties and recognising what a massive achievement it can be to keep your head above water while caring for children. It is also understanding where we are being let down because of, for instance, low pay, insecure work or shoddy housing.

We should not discount maternal care and love because it does not fit narrow, morally based conceptions of child development. The dignity of motherdom means valuing all that mothers do for their children.

Motherdom Is Not Telling Mothers What to Do

Expert advice which instructs mothers what to do infantilises them. It can also undermine other valuable sources of guidance, such as friends, siblings, parents and grandparents (expert advice can be particularly dismissive of the knowledge and experience of older generations). Motherdom incorporates multiple sources of information and wisdom. Expert knowledge should be part of the constellation of influences to take into account when making decisions.

Anyone who writes the words 'informed choice' should stop and think about what they are really trying to do and how realistic it is. Public health messaging should be achievable and not set women up to fail. If it isn't working, the onus should be on asking why that is – and looking to change those wider factors for the better rather than piling emotional pressure onto women.

Breastfeeding is a really good example of this. Women are told how important breastfeeding is, but they are not provided with adequate feeding support and the factors that make breastfeeding challenging are ignored. It is too easy to assume that women are not breastfeeding because of a lack of knowledge. The solution is then to 'inform' women, instead of providing them with practical help if they want to breastfeed, and respecting their decision if they don't.

This would require a huge cultural and political shift, but instead of telling mothers what to do, we should listen to them instead. They are experts in their children. Women bringing up children in challenging circumstances, such as surviving on low incomes and living in unsafe neighbourhoods, understand how to mother in those contexts. As we explored in Chapter 1, Jennifer Randles's term 'inventive mothering' conveys the resourcefulness and ingenuity employed by women in tackling the difficulties they encounter.[14]

The work of the sociologist Priya Fielding-Singh illuminates the dynamics shaping decision-making with a richness and compassion which I wish we could find in all research on mothers. For low-income parents, allowing their children to have junk food is about 'honoring and nurturing', an opportunity to say yes to their children's wishes when poverty so often means they have to say no. Time-pressed mothers, working in physically taxing jobs such as cleaning, have precious little energy or time for cooking. More convenient and less healthy options therefore make more sense. Fielding-Singh writes: 'Choices that may have seemed strange from the outside revealed themselves to me as perfectly reasonable and rational.'[15]

Policymakers should recognise the value of parents' experiences and views. Mothers' perspectives must be sought out and prioritised (those of other parents and caregivers too). It should never be assumed that needs are universal – diverse groups of people need to be around the table. As I have explored in this book, expert advice often ignores the daily reality of women's lives. The historian Ellen Ross recounts that around the turn of the twentieth century, middle-class officials urged working-class mothers to feed their children porridge. This disregarded the fact that poorer families could not afford the milk and had few cooking pots. These pots retained the odour of previous meals, making the porridge taste revolting.[16] Instead of telling women to make porridge, it would have been better to ask families what they needed to feed children nutritiously. Having enough money to buy food would be a good start.

Motherdom Means Understanding and Supporting Other Mothers

Women together can challenge Good Mother myths. The writer and social worker Kelly Jeske puts it magnificently:

> When mothers zip up, suit up, and put masks over our pain and uncertainty, we contribute to the silencing and erasure of other mothers . . . It could be so different: mothers speaking our truths as we live them – sharing our strengths and our fears, our misses and our triumphs. Allowing ourselves imperfection and rawness and uncertainty.[17]

But the binds, constraints and oppression suffered by some mothers can be invisible or ignored by women who are privileged by class, race, health or sexuality. It is important to appreciate the different burdens that mothers carry and how these can be multiplied by different forms of disadvantage. In a 1980 conference paper, Audre Lorde argued that women must recognise each other's differences 'to enrich our visions and our joint struggles':

> Some problems we share as women, some we do not. You fear your children will grow up to join the patriarchy and testify against you, we fear our children will be dragged from a car and shot down in the street, and you will turn your backs upon the reasons they are dying.[18]

We must all commit to listening and understanding better. This can also help us be more honest ourselves. Our starting assumption should be, until we have good reason to think otherwise, that each mother we come across loves her children and is trying to do the best she can in her particular circumstances.

We cannot let Good Mother myths poison our discussions and interactions with other parents. The concept of 'optimal' makes disagreements inevitable. Because child-rearing practices are inherently variable, there are very few definitively 'right' answers. But the pressure to provide the 'best' care means that women find themselves having to justify their decisions. Science and nature are called upon to referee discussions such as whether babies should sleep on their own or in bed with parents. In their research on online communities, the academics Jessica Clements and Kari Nixon describe how 'mothers in social media mothering groups fling data back and forth at one another like weapons . . . demonstrating a remarkable ability to critique study design only when it suits them, for the argument was never about data to begin with – it was about self-worth and validity'.[19]

We need to recognise when our personal moral outrage towards mothers has been triggered – why is this and how fair are we being? In her piece 'I Was a Screen-Time Expert. Then the Coronavirus Happened', the writer Anya Kamenetz apologised to anyone who 'felt judged or shamed by my, or anyone's, implication that they weren't good parents because they weren't successfully enforcing a "healthy balance" with screens, either for themselves or their children. That was a fat honking wad of privilege speaking.'[20]

To temper our moral outrage, it can be salutary to consider what lies behind maternal practices that affront us in some way. One thing I have learned from my work with new mothers is that there is always a reason why women are doing, saying or feeling something. The rationale may sound awkward and forced because of the narrow constraints of acceptability in which women have to operate, like a woman saying that her newborn baby likes their own space to justify why she isn't interacting with the baby during every waking moment.

Sharing experiences and perspectives with other mothers is a powerful antidote to Good Mother myths. As the writer Rebecca Solnit observes, 'Liberation is always in part a storytelling process: breaking stories, breaking silences, making new stories.'[21] Digital spaces have opened up new opportunities for mothers to do this. The sociologist Tina Miller researched the experience of becoming a mother in the late 1990s and then did a similar study two decades later. She observes that while mothering is still 'intensified, individualised and . . . undervalued', women now have access to 'a wider, digitally available spectrum of maternal experiences'.[22]

However, as Clements and Nixon note, these digital spaces can be 'formed around polarities (e.g., formula vs. breastfeeding groups, co-sleeping vs. safe sleeping groups) rather than unifying factors'. These positions are then enforced 'by aggressive and systematic meme sharing and message-board vigilantism'. This perpetuates rather than challenges Good Mother myths.

The value of open and honest discussions is a common thread running through research studies among mothers. For instance, a US qualitative study asked African American and Latina mothers to make recommendations to health providers working with new mothers living with postpartum depression. They suggested getting women together to share their experiences: 'It helps a lot to see that you are not the only one who is going through that.'[23] When I was sorting through my mum's papers after she died, I found a research report she had written in 1981 for her local health authority, 'Post-Natal Groups – Is There a Need?' On the basis of the survey, which she carried out with fifty-one women and her discussions with new mothers, she concluded that there was. She recommended that the groups be run by health visitors but 'ideally it would be the mothers helping with and discussing problems for themselves, with little professional intervention'.

At the end of every postnatal course I have run, the women say how much they have appreciated being able to talk openly to others in the same boat. Hearing other mothers are experiencing similar problems and emotions shifts the focus from self-blame to a broader and more productive canvas. It can be hugely beneficial to discuss the day-to-day practices of mothering in arenas which are not policed by Good Mother myths. We can learn a lot from other people, benefiting from what Clements and Nixon call 'collective knowledge creation'. Sharing our predicaments with others can give us practical solutions, different perspectives or reassurance that others are experiencing the same things.

In addition, observing the myriad different ways that other women mother illustrates that there is no one right way. The spectre of the Good Mother is banished. Motherhood is deeply rooted in our personal and social context – 'plural and specific to time and place and situation' as the historian Sarah Knott puts it.[24] There are few easy answers, and part of the endeavour of child-rearing is thoughtful consideration of our actions and decisions.

Motherdom Encompasses Ambivalence, Contradictions and Regrets

'The experience shared variously by all mothers in which loving and hating feelings for their children exist side by side' is how the psychotherapist Rozsika Parker defines maternal ambivalence.[25] Parker and the psychiatrist and psychoanalyst Barbara Almond both argue that mothers need to come to terms with maternal ambivalence as part of their emotional lives. This ambivalence can be manageable or unmanageable, but we cannot wish it away. Like all relationships, our relationship with our children can be joyful and fulfilling, as well as complicated, frustrating and difficult. But profound feelings of love, a deep sense of responsibility and children's reliance on their caregivers makes this relationship especially intense and complex.

Almond counsels against trying to mask ambivalence through performance art as the 'too good mother' who is determined to do everything right.[26] This can increase the burden of Good Mother myths. In a UK study among women experiencing post-natal depression, the researchers suggested that depressed mothers may have similar thoughts and feelings as other mothers but have more difficulty accepting their ambivalent feelings.[27]

Maternal ambivalence can be productive – even 'transformative' in Parker's words – when it leads to women thinking creatively about how to deal with their difficulties mothering. Parker argues: 'A mother needs to know herself, to own up to the diverse, contradictory, often overwhelming feelings evoked by motherhood . . . It's only by accepting that at times you are a bad mother, that you can ever be a good mother.'[28]

Motherdom means accepting ambivalence and, related to this, the contradictions of motherhood. One of these is how we can lose ourselves in our children at the same time as learning new things about ourselves. Another is our conflicting emotions. Raising children can be relentless and sublime and boring and joyful and energising and draining all at the same time. It is normal to love our children but to find the day-to-day tasks of parenting, like playing and bathing, tedious some or all of the time. Children can seem charming, mesmerising and beautiful one minute, annoying, whingey and demanding the next. Child-rearing can be very hard work. Love and frustration intermingle. No one has infuriated or worried me like my children have, but no one else has been the source of so much delight either. I have watched them grow with pride and amazement and learned so much about the world from them.

Motherdom is also about regrets. This is different from guilt and shame, which can be very toxic. Guilt directs our attention inwards to our apparent inadequacies, rather than looking outwards and realising how we and our children are being failed. As the psychologist Harriet Lerner has observed, 'our society encourages mothers to cultivate guilt like a little flower garden . . . Guilt keeps mothers narrowly focused on the question, "What's wrong with me?" and prevents us from becoming effective agents of personal and social change.'[29]

'Poignant regrets' is a phrase that Joan Raphael-Leff uses which resonates deeply for me. She observed that such regrets are 'part and parcel of the difficult emotional task of every thoughtful mother who finds that reality can never be as perfect as she would like it for her infant'.[30] I have many poignant regrets when I contemplate my mothering over the years.

'I know I made mistakes', the feminist writer and activist Lynne Segal reflects in *Lean on Me: A Politics of Radical Care*. She raised her son in a communal household shared with two other single mothers and 'always a few men'. She and her son flourished in this 'laid-back, uncompetitive, extremely permissive atmosphere', and he recalls his childhood as 'wonderful'. However, Segal also feels she did not adequately prepare her son for a driven and competitive world and wonders whether she should have offered him more of her 'overriding personal focus'.[31] As Segal's reflections illustrate, we can give our children a splendid childhood but still question whether we could have done things differently.

I believe regrets are an inescapable part of loving children. Because we care so deeply for them, we don't want to get things wrong or harm them. But it is inevitable we will make mistakes, some small, some big. We may try to avoid the blunders and wrongs of our parents, but we have our own foibles and blind spots. We bring so much emotional baggage to motherhood: past and present anxieties, suffering and trauma. Sometimes we may need help dealing with our pain and the heavy weight of the past, both for our sake and our children's.

Motherdom entails accepting that we are flawed – but also that children do not need perfection. If we try and be perfect, we can lose sight of ourselves and our children. And our children are imperfect humans too. They deserve to be loved, regardless.

Motherdom Is Selfhood

Selfhood outside of motherhood is an essential element of motherdom. The value of mothers as people in their own right must be recognised and respected.

Motherdom is not martyrdom. Motherhood should not be about self-sacrifice and the obliteration of self. A mother is still a person, with valid needs, fears and hopes. In her essay 'The Impossibility of the Good Black Mother', the writer T. F. Charlton emphasises the need to:

See worth and dignity in the beautiful mess of singularities and complexities that we are. This is better than being acknowledged as a Good Mother: to be seen as a mother and fully human at once. This is liberation.[32]

Motherdom involves sustaining both our and our children's selfhood. We are interdependent but also separate, and this dynamic oscillates over time and according to context. How we feel about this can fluctuate a great deal too. Babies are intensely dependent on their caregivers, and some women adore this phase, while others find it overwhelming and claustrophobic. They may instead relish being the mother of an energetic toddler, full of questions and curiosity. For others, the constant activity and talking can drive them to distraction. Equally, the teenage years can bring enjoyment of a child's burgeoning independence or feel like painful rejection.

The writer Chimamanda Ngozi Adichie advises mothers: 'Be a full person. Motherhood is a glorious gift, but do not define yourself solely by motherhood. Be a full person. Your child will benefit from that.'[33] Selfhood matters not just for us but for our children too. Part of the job of parents is preparing our children for the world. Being a full person helps children understand that other people have needs and wishes. The self-sacrificing, self-abnegating mother who is constantly responsive to her children provides an unrealistic and unhelpful model of human relationships. Our daughters absorb norms that women are givers, while our sons may become accultured to the role of taker. I feel lucky to have grown up with a mother who had a job that she found meaningful and who loved to become engrossed in sewing or reading. She inspired me in many ways (although I never managed to learn to sew).

We need to consider and value all the bonds that children have. Focusing solely on mothers is not good for women or for children. Other family members – not just fathers but also grandparents, step-parents, aunts, uncles, siblings – matter too. Then there are significant others who can be a powerful influence on children (for good or for ill), such as friends, teachers and people in the neighbourhood. Children's development and wellbeing should be seen in the context of a web of relationships of varying closeness and supportiveness. Alison Gopnik highlights that children learn 'from observing and imitating many different kinds of people with different skills . . . by listening to many different kinds of people talking about many different kinds of things in different kinds of ways'.[34]

There can be an understandable resistance to this from mothers. bell hooks has observed in feminist thought an 'unwillingness to concede motherhood as an arena of social life in which women can exert power and control'.[35] I think we can say that motherhood is special because the work of bringing up children is valuable and important. But, at the same time, responsibility for child-rearing is open to everyone and is not solely the domain of women. As Andrea O'Reilly argues, this makes empowered mothering possible because it 'allows a woman selfhood outside of motherhood and affords her power within motherhood'.[36]

Motherdom Involves Calling Bullshit on the Myth of the Natural and Bad Science

Mary Wollstonecraft described advice on women's behaviour as 'specious poisons' which are 'strenuously inculcated' in women.[37] We need to spurn the specious poisons which underpin Good Mother myths.

The myth of the natural is a toxin which is used to judge, control and devalue women. However, this myth doesn't stand up to any meaningful scrutiny. A cursory glance across time, geography and culture shows us how much variation there is in maternal care. As the anthropologist Nancy Scheper-Hughes argues: 'Mother love is anything *other* than natural and instead represents a matrix of images, meanings, sentiments, and practices that are everywhere socially and culturally produced.' In her work living among and studying families in a Brazilian shanty town, she observed how women's experiences of multiple child deaths meant that 'mother love grows slowly, tentatively, and fearfully'.[38] To adapt Simone de Beauvoir's celebrated rejection of biological essentialism – one is not born, but rather becomes, a mother.[39]

Shaky science is the source of much specious poison. It helps fuel mother blame and prescribes how women should behave and feel in relation to their children. Attachment theory and brain claims are infused with magical thinking and deeply entrenched assumptions that women can and should sacrifice everything in their power for their children. And even this is not enough – the current orthodoxy of 'the more the better' means that women will always fall short.

Attachment research is distorted to hold women responsible for how their children turn out and to instruct them to be 'sensitive'. Neuroscience is used to justify detailed prescriptions such as 'serve and return'. We must call out magical thinking on both. Attempting to micromanage interactions between mothers and their children devalues the many different ways women care for their children and show their love. It is such a narrow and dismal notion of mothering, and loving kids because it is good for their brains is a particularly bleak view of human relationships.

Science both mirrors and powers mother blame. Good Mother myths will endure if we don't tackle the use and abuse of science in telling women what to do. Poorly conducted and misinterpreted science is a problem for society in general, not just mothers. Dorothy Bishop, the champion of robust science who featured in Chapter 2, argues that failing to challenge bad science allows 'wrongheaded interventions or policies' which can 'damage the wellbeing of individuals or society', as well as letting down future generations who are trying to build on a research base lacking solid foundations. Bad science is harmful in so many ways.[40]

Bishop advocates aligning research incentives with efforts to counteract flawed science, with researchers rewarded for doing replicable research.[41] She also favours having safeguards in place to prevent the cherry-picking of evidence. The American Statistical Association vigorously counsels against significance chasing and recommends transparency to avoid the temptation to do so: 'Researchers should disclose the number of hypotheses explored during the study, all data collection decisions, all statistical analyses conducted, and all p-values computed.'[42]

Transparency is key to good science. This makes any attempts to slice and dice data to prove pre-existing assumptions much more obvious. One specific area where I would like to see more information is sample sizes. How many people are in the sample and what are the numbers in subgroup analysis (information which was not disclosed in the mother-love-brain-size studies we looked at in Chapter 2)? I was drilled from the start of my research career on the importance of including all sample sizes when reporting data, and I find the failure of papers published in respectable journals to do so absolutely baffling.

Another important area where there is a lack of transparency is how overall measures used in studies have been developed and defined. Without being able to see under the bonnet, we don't know what is actually being measured and what sort of value judgements are at play. Because the Maternal Behaviour Q-Sort, a well-known way of measuring sensitivity which was discussed in Chapter 5, has been published we can appraise the sweeping value judgements it makes. As we saw, it is apparently insensitive to stop interacting with the baby if the telephone rings or to use a 'sibling or television' to keep the baby entertained.

Transparency in research is also about making background assumptions visible. To draw on Helen Longino's thinking once again, these assumptions should be articulated so they can be subjected to criticism and then 'defended, modified, or abandoned in response to such criticism'. As Longino points out, concealing background assumptions discourages the investigation of alternative frameworks.[43] Any assumption that child development is predominantly driven by maternal behaviour should be stated outright.

I think we need to ditch this background assumption in any case. The design of research studies should be based on a wide-ranging conception of children's development instead of focusing on the minutiae of maternal care. Otherwise, the research is context-free and fails to ask the relevant questions. It leads to circular reasoning because focusing solely on the mother–child relationship means that how children develop is then attributed to what mothers do or don't do. Conclusions will, inevitably, be narrow, leading us down blind alleys such as sensitivity training – when the bigger problem is that mothers don't have enough money to pay the bills.

Press releases are another important issue to tackle. These are a major problem leading to simplistic and inaccurate claims. This is not good for the reputation of science in the long term. The fact-checking charity Full Fact has called for university, charity and think tank press offices to issue accurate press releases. This requires including all important caveats, links to source material and only using quotes that accurately represent the research.[44] I think these rules should also apply to policy reports which package up research evidence. As we've seen, these can wildly misrepresent the evidence and perpetuate a culture of mother blame. We need to jettison flimsy brain claims and alarmist contentions about corrosive cortisol.

It must always be made clear in any press release or report when a study being cited has not been carried out on people. Say when it is animal research. Using animal studies to make points about human relationships without saying so explicitly is dishonest and unethical. People can then come to their own conclusions about whether they should listen to edicts issued on the basis of research done with rats.

I would also like to see more detailed, immersive studies like those done by Priya Fielding-Singh and Nancy Scheper-Hughes. Research about families should also encompass participatory methods, enabling parents and children to shape what is researched and how the findings are used.[45] This would give us a far richer understanding of families than laboratory tasks, brain scans and spurious correlations.

Motherdom Means Creating a Better Society

Motherdom, I believe, should encompass a broader and more constructive understanding of what children need to thrive. We must turn away from mother blame and stop laying responsibility for children's lives at the feet of mothers. Instead, our starting point should be to assume that mothers (and fathers and other caregivers) want to do what's best for their children – what is getting in the way? It is a long and daunting list: poverty, racism, pollution, inadequate housing, low wages, insecure jobs, poor healthcare and food insecurity.

Babies and children are among the most vulnerable members of society, deserving of love and security, as well as necessities such as good nutrition and somewhere safe to live. Giving children a good start in life is a moral imperative. It should be a matter of deep public shame that in wealthy countries like the UK and the US there are children who don't have enough to eat, who have to live in overcrowded, damp, mouldy, vermin-infested homes with no heating or hot water. In both countries, children have to go to sleep at night on empty stomachs. A World Vision/Ipsos survey found that 18% of parents in the US and 14% in the UK said that a child in their household had gone to bed hungry in the last thirty days because of a lack of food.[46]

Children deserve to live in safe neighbourhoods with clean air and places to play. Families have a right to expect decent housing, good education, access to healthcare and affordable transport to school, work and shops. Public spaces like parks, sports facilities and libraries are beneficial for everyone. These are places for families to enjoy and which bring people together.

In the US, guns are a scourge for families. Writer and activist Mikki Kendall argues persuasively that gun violence is a feminist issue, not just because of gun-related domestic violence but also because guns make homes, schools and streets unsafe for American children, with Black children and teens most at risk.[47]

Children and their parents must be protected from intimate partner violence, a blight on the lives of everyone involved. Shelters and support for victims of violence and their children should be a public health priority. A double bind is that women are supposed to shield their children from domestic violence, but they and their relationships with their children are not protected. Perpetrators can deploy a range of tactics to undermine the mother–child relationship, such as insults, criticisms, jealousy and threats to report the woman to child protection services. They may even try to destroy the relationship altogether through homicide or abduction.[48]

Child welfare needs to be overhauled. Dorothy Roberts makes a powerful case for dismantling the current child welfare system in the US: 'We need to build a safer society by reimagining the very meaning of child welfare and protection and by creating caring ways of supporting families and meeting children's needs.'[49] Brid Featherstone, Anna Gupta, Kate Morris and Sue White make similar arguments for the UK in *Protecting Children: A Social Model*: '"Child protection" needs to be remade fundamentally in the interests of protecting children and building a good society for them and those who care for, and about, them.'[50]

Unmothering must be a last resort. It is unforgivable that babies and children are removed from their mothers because of a cocktail of bogus brain claims, poverty and insufficient support. The heartbreaking testimonies of parents and children in the forced adoption scandals warn us of the profound and lifelong pain that can be inflicted.

Work and childcare are fundamental to rethinking motherhood. Jobs need to be more secure, better paid, more flexible and free from harassment and discrimination. These protections should be for everyone, including migrants and lower-paid workers. This would be widely beneficial – greater economic security and the opportunity to spend more time outside work would be advantageous for everyone, not just parents.

A new model of work with policies to support working parents would enable men to get more involved in childcare and labour at home. The sociologist Caitlyn Collins terms this 'work-family justice' – 'a system in which each member of society has the opportunity and power to fully participate in both paid work and family care'.[51]

A key requirement for making employment work for parents is universal, high-quality and affordable childcare. There are economic arguments for subsidising day care because increasing labour participation generates tax revenue and reduces welfare payments.[52] It can also benefit children. There is good evidence from two longitudinal studies, one conducted in England and one in the US, that high-quality pre-school care can have a positive long-term impact on children's educational attainment and behaviour and can lessen the negative impact of poverty.[53]

It is stating the obvious to say that society cannot function without care work – caring for children, the elderly and the sick, cooking, cleaning, washing and shopping. Yet this work is not properly valued or remunerated. It is instead offloaded to the poorly paid and powerless and is often underfunded and invisible. As Caroline Criado Perez rightly argues, the exclusion of care services from the general concept of infrastructure 'is just another unquestioned male bias in how we structure our economy'.[54]

Creating a 'caring economy' has been advocated by the Commission on a Gender-Equal Economy established by the UK Women's Budget Group. Central to this is investment in social infrastructure – that is to say healthcare, social care, education services, universal childcare provision, specialist violence against women and girls support providers, affordable housing and high-quality public transport.[55] I'd add here that investment in healthcare must include properly resourced maternity services and postnatal care, including feeding support. Otherwise we cannot meaningfully address the problems with feeding and birth discussed in Chapters 3 and 4.

Another specific element of social infrastructure to highlight is early years work. It is important and deserves more respect and better pay. In the UK, the workforce is traditionally female and on low rates of pay.[56] In the US, early years workers are also low-income, predominantly female and disproportionately women of colour, reflecting longstanding patterns of occupational segregation and racial discrimination.[57] If the sector had more prestige and better pay, this would encourage more male employees. bell hooks argues persuasively that male childcare workers can 'help promote awareness of the necessity for male participation in childraising'.[58]

Motherdom Requires Reproductive Justice

Social infrastructure needs to be underpinned by a framework of reproductive justice, a concept invented by Black women in 1994, which combines reproductive rights and social justice. This places these rights in a political context which highlights that access, power and resources are determined by race and class. Reproductive justice recognises the right to maintain personal bodily autonomy, to have children, to not have children and to raise children with dignity in safe, healthy and supportive environments.[59] We are so far off that now.

The overturning of Roe v. Wade, the 1973 Supreme Court judgement protecting the right to have an abortion, signals frightening times ahead for reproductive rights in the United States. It is not just about denying the right to abortion, devastating though that is. We may also be entering a new era of unmothering. The Supreme Court judgement overturning Roe quotes a 2008 report about the virtually non-existent 'domestic supply of infants' for adoption and cites arguments that 'a woman who puts her newborn up for adoption today has little reason to fear that the baby will not find a suitable home.'[60] The implications of this are chilling: babies routinely taken away from 'Bad Mothers' to give them to 'deserving' families.

Anyone who cares about babies and children should care about reproductive rights. As Sarah Hrdy argues, infanticide, abandonment and wet nursing are only unthinkable in societies where women have reproductive control or can share childcare.[61]

A rights discourse will also mean that debates and deliberations on birth, feeding and child-rearing can be much more productively framed. If we start with the assumption that mothers and birthing people are human beings of worth and autonomy, the double binds which can be so damaging begin to melt away.

Our Own Personal Motherdom

I will end with a consideration of what motherdom means on a personal level. This is my individual take, and others will have different views and experiences. The concept of motherdom is flexible enough to incorporate many perspectives.

My starting point is that our own personal motherdom means doing what works for us and our families in the here and now. Our mothering is shaped by so many factors: our personalities, values, childhood experiences, cultural heritage, income, work, health, levels of social support and family situation. Because of all of this, some elements of caregiving may come easily, while others are difficult or frustrating. It is ok to throw ourselves into the bits of parenting we enjoy and try to avoid those that we don't. We can leave those parts of caregiving to someone else where possible or perhaps just not do them at all. Imaginary play, for example, can feel awkward and tedious to an adult. Children do not need adults to play, and for most of human history, children have been left to play by themselves.

When we spend time with our children, we can instead find ways to involve them in what interests us or look for things to do that everyone enjoys. We should banish anxieties about adequately stimulating and entertaining them. These get in the way of enjoying the here and now with our children. Mothers should trust that they are enough, that their love and attention are precious to their children (even the teenagers who push them away).

Individual motherdom also means mothering in a way that suits the children we have. There is so much variation in children's personalities and needs. My two children are very distinct people, and this was apparent from birth. One fell upon dummies with delight, while the other spat the dummy across the room in disgust. They are teenagers now and how we connect (and what we argue about) is very particular to each of them.

There are many dilemmas to face in raising children. Questions such as when to intervene and when to stand back have no definitive or easy answers. I have often recommended the 'misery test' to new mothers in my postnatal work. If something is making us or our children feel miserable or stressed, take that as a signal to reconsider or do something different. I have found it a good rule of thumb. As I have said, mistakes and poignant regrets are inevitable, but they can teach us something too. Motherdom is a realm where we continue to learn as our children grow and change (and we do too).

Much of what we are told about mothers and attachment theory is bollocks. But the secure base and safe haven of attachment theory are powerful concepts. This means being a person a child can count on when it matters – someone who provides a secure base which allows them to explore the world and a safe haven to turn to when they need comfort or protection.

How this secure base and safe haven works will be deeply personal and also highly circumstantial. Comforting an ill toddler is different from consoling a pre-teen who has just fallen out with their best friend. But the contours of comfort can endure as our children get older. I was reminded of this recently when I was in hospital with one of my children. As we talked to each other, they absent-mindedly played with the scarf I was wearing. It took me back to when my child was small and would gently tug the ends of my scarf as we walked alongside each other. That scarf, then and now, signifies that we are both interdependent and separate.

Sometimes we long to put things right for our children but we can't. The domain of motherdom can only go so far. We are unable to stop our colicky baby from crying, magic away the shattering medical diagnosis our child has just received or mend our teenager's broken heart. But what we can do is provide a safe haven by being there with them and for them. I think this is one of the very hardest parts of motherhood, accepting how little power we really have to shape our children's lives. We can make a difference to their happiness – and mothers have the power to make their children very unhappy – but we cannot change who they are or many of the things that will happen to them.

Although there are no guarantees, the one thing we can definitely control is our love and acceptance of our children. They have their own needs, hopes, desires and ambitions. I think it is important to maintain a sense of curiosity about our children, about who they are and what they care about. This may be very different to what we expected or wanted. I believe that is ok as long as *they* are ok.

We should put our personal motherdom in a wider context; mothers cannot do it alone. It is everyone's responsibility to provide a nurturing, safe and equitable garden for children to grow into adults. At the same time, we should all celebrate the love and care and toil and endeavour which mothers so generously give.

Acknowledgements

I owe a deep debt of gratitude to the work of many writers and researchers. I hope I have done them justice in these pages. I'd like to thank Andrea O'Reilly and the Centre for Parenting Culture Studies at the University of Kent for helping me discover reams of interesting material about motherhood.

A massive thank you to Leo Hollis, who has very generously shared his time and wisdom with me. I'm grateful to Poppy Hampson, who also helped me tackle the daunting world of publishing. A big thank you to David Lynch and Fen Starkey for your feedback on my book proposal.

Many thanks to my wonderful agent Eleanor Birne. I hugely appreciate you championing this book and helping me to get it out into the world. Thank you as well to the rest of the team at PEW Literary. Cora MacGregor came up with the excellent title, Patrick Walsh was a huge help in finessing my book proposal and Charlotte van Wijk gave me faith that this is a book with important things to say.

I am so grateful to my brilliant editor Rosie Warren, who has been a joy to work with. This book is all the better for your keen insights, astute suggestions and wise editing. I'd also like to thank everyone else at Verso, especially Nick Walther and Melissa Weiss, for their help with the text and the cover, and Maya Osborne for publicity.

My thinking, and my world in general, have been enhanced by treasured friends who entered my life at different stages. I'm listing you in chronological and alphabetical order. From the school and Bath days: Adele Hudson, Alice Wynne-Edwards, Cath Sainsbury, Fen Starkey, Hayley Spooner, Karyn von Engelbrechten, Kath Roper,

Lindsay Hawdon, Maria Cadenas, Sarah Dakin, Sophie Knock, Susie Moss and Toria Roper. From university and the Approach Road era: Dave Cunnington, Edmund Moriarty, Esther Perez, Jane Fearn, Janet Bradley, John Edwards, Jon Harwood, Kamlesh Gupta, Luke Jacobs, Martin Kearton, Nadine Winkler, Phil Luther, Ray Winkler, Sandy Maudgil, Sarah Prietzsch and Steve Ballinger. From the MORI times: Annabelle Phillips, Ben Page, Billie Ing, Jo Down, Kirsten Colley, Pauline McGowan, Rebecca Klahr, Renata Apostolaki, Sara Grant-Vest and Suzanne Hall. And the mothering years: Anna Richardson, Ceri Fuller, Fatema Sardharwala, Hetal Patel, Lisa Moran Parker, Liz Day, Lucy Sandeberg, Mary Burrows, Miranda Rosenthal, Pandora Clifford, Penny Seguss, Roo Tindall, Sally Randall and Sian Sargaison.

A very special thank you to Lindsay Hawdon, from whom I have learnt so much about writing, mothering and life, and to Anna Richardson, who has had my back in the motherdom trenches from day one.

I'd like to say thank you to all the NCT practitioners, staff and Clapham volunteers who I have talked with and learned from over the years. A special shout-out to my fellow postnatal practitioners: you are awesome. Many thanks to Mary Newburn for guiding me through a research overview on the transition to motherhood and to Abigail Easter for explaining cortisol to me.

An enormous thank you to my family: my father, Andrew, my brother, James, my stepmother, Pat, my stepsiblings, Ruth and Kevin and the fabulous Farrziz. Thank you to my in-laws, Di, Daniel, Beany and Paul, for welcoming me into your family.

I am immensely grateful to my husband, Chris, for everything, not least being so supportive of my 'booking' (in his words). I forgive you for getting your book published before mine. Especial thanks to my precious children, Orson and Juno, who have shaped this book and enriched my life.

My final thanks must go to my beloved mother, Pamela Cumming. If she were still here, I know she would be buttonholing everyone she met to tell them about this book. I miss her beyond words.

Notes

Introduction

1. N. Stadlen (2004). *What Mothers Do: Especially When It Looks Like Nothing*. Piatkus.
2. A. Rich (1986). *Of Woman Born: Motherhood as Experience and Institution* (2nd ed.). W. W. Norton & Company.
3. Ibid.
4. J. Rose (2018). *Mothers: An Essay on Love and Cruelty*. Faber & Faber.
5. D. P. Moynihan (1965). *The Moynihan Report: The Negro Family – The Case for National Action*. United States Department of Labor.
6. R. A. Spitz & W. G. Cobliner (1965). *The First Year of Life: A Psychoanalytic Study of Normal and Deviant Development of Object Relations*. International Universities Press.
7. Quoted in H. A. Washington (2006). *Medical Apartheid: The Dark History of Medical Experimentation on Black Americans from Colonial Times to the Present*. Anchor Books.
8. D. Ockenden (2020). *Emerging Findings and Recommendations from the Independent Review of Maternity Services at the Shrewsbury and Telford Hospital NHS Trust*. HC 1081.
9. Quoted in T. Jensen (2018). *Parenting the Crisis: The Cultural Politics of Parent-Blame*. Policy Press.
10. S. Maitland (1980). Untitled. In S. Dowrick & S. Grundberg. *Why Children?* (78–91). The Women's Press.
11. K. Manne (2019). *Down Girl: The Logic of Misogyny*. Penguin Books.
12. S. Hustvedt (2021). *Mothers, Fathers, and Others: New Essays*. Sceptre.
13. S. Heti (2018). *Motherhood*. Harvill Secker.
14. M. West, R. Kraut & H. E. Chew (2019). *I'd Blush If I Could: Closing Gender divides in Digital skills through Education*. EQUALS and UNESCO.

15. J. Roberts-Crews (2020, 15 May). Resisting Mammy Professorhood During COVID-19. *Medium*.
16. Rose, 2018.
17. S. Federici (1975). *Wages Against Housework*. Falling Wall Press.
18. A. McClintock (1995). *Imperial Leather: Race, Gender, and Sexuality in the Colonial Contest*. Routledge.
19. H. Wentworth (1941). The Allegedly Dead Suffix -dom in Modern English. *PMLA*, 56(1), 280–306.

1. Good Mother Myths at Work

1. A. Combe & J. Clark (1860). *The Management of Infancy: Physiological and Moral*. Kessinger Legacy Reprints.
2. A. Davin (1978). Imperialism and Motherhood. *History Workshop, 5*, 9–65.
3. J. Lewis (1980). *The Politics of Motherhood: Child and Maternal Welfare in England, 1900–1939*. McGill-Queen's Press.
4. Quoted in M. Ladd-Taylor (1994). *Mother-Work: Women, Child Welfare, and the State, 1890–1930*. University of Illinois Press.
5. M. Alsan & C. Goldin (2019). Watersheds in Child Mortality: The Role of Effective Water and Sewerage Infrastructure, 1880–1920. *Journal of Political Economy*, 127(2), 586–638. P. J. Atkins (2003). Mother's Milk and Infant Death in Britain, circa 1900–1940. *Anthropology of Food*, (2).
6. E. Pritchard (1921). *The Infant: Nutrition and Management* (2nd ed.). Edward Arnold.
7. C. Urwin & E. Sharland (1992). From Bodies to Minds in Childcare Literature: Advice to Parents in Inter-War Britain. In R. Cooter (Ed.). *In the Name of the Child: Health and Welfare, 1880–1940* (174–99). Routledge.
8. Davin, 1978.
9. J. Golden (2018). *Babies Made Us Modern: How Infants Brought America into the Twentieth Century*. Cambridge University Press.
10. F. Truby-King (1913). *Feeding and Care of Baby*. Macmillan and Co.
11. E. Ross (1993). *Love and Toil: Motherhood in Outcast London, 1870–1918*. Oxford University Press.
12. Pritchard, 1921.
13. J. B. Watson (1928). Against the Threat of Mother Love. Reprinted in H. Jenkins (Ed.). *Childhood in Contemporary Cultures* (470–5). New York University Press.
14. Ross, 1993; Lewis, 1980.
15. Golden, 2018.
16. Urwin & Sharland, 1992.

17. M. Hogarth (1935). Development of the Child: 2 to 14. In G. St Aubyn (Ed.). *The Family Book: A Comprehensive Guide – Primarily for Parents* (427–52). Arthur Barker.

18. P. N. Stearns (2015). Childhood Emotions in Modern Western History. In P. S. Fass (Ed.). *The Routledge History of Childhood in the Western World* (158–73). Routledge.

19. Committee for the Study of the Future of Public Health (1988). *The Future of Public Health*. National Academies Press.

20. Alsan & Goldin, 2019.

21. A. Bhatia, N. Krieger & S. V. Subramanian (2019). Learning from History About Reducing Infant Mortality: Contrasting the Centrality of Structural Interventions to Early 20th-Century Successes in the United States to Their Neglect in Current Global Initiatives. *The Milbank Quarterly*, 97(1), 285–345. R. I. Woods, P. A. Watterson & J. H. Woodward (1989). The Causes of Rapid Infant Mortality Decline in England and Wales, 1861–1921. Part II. *Population Studies*, 43(1), 113–32.

22. Lewis, 1980.

23. S. Lassonde (2015). Age, Schooling, and Development. In P. S. Fass (Ed.). *The Routledge History of Childhood in the Western World* (211–28). Routledge.

24. A. Turmel (2008). *A Historical Sociology of Childhood: Developmental Thinking, Categorisation and Graphic Visualisation*. Cambridge University Press.

25. D. T. Cook (2015). Children as Consumers: History and Histography. In P. S. Fass (Ed.). *The Routledge History of Childhood in the Western World* (283–95). Routledge.

26. S. Frankenburg (1922). *Common Sense in the Nursery*. Christophers; S. Frankenburg (1946). *Common Sense in the Nursery* (3rd ed.). Penguin.

27. C. A. Aldrich & M. M. Aldrich (1938). *Babies Are Human Beings: An Interpretation of Growth*. The Macmillan Company.

28. Urwin & Sharland, 1992.

29. Golden, 2018.

30. A. Davis (2012). *Modern Motherhood: Women and Family in England, 1945–2000*. Manchester University Press.

31. R. D. Apple (2006). *Perfect Motherhood: Science and Childrearing in America*. Rutgers University Press.

32. T. Maier (1998). *Dr Spock: An American Life*. Harcourt Brace.

33. B. Spock (1946). *The Common Sense Book of Baby and Child Care*. Duell, Sloan and Pearce.

34. Maier, 1998.

35. B. Spock & M. Morgan (1985). *Spock on Spock: A Memoir of Growing up with the Century*. Pantheon Books.

36. B. Spock (1976). *Baby & Child Care*. Pocket Books.

37. J. Vandenberg-Daves (2014). *Modern Motherhood: An American History*. Rutgers University Press.

38. F. Lundberg & M. F. Farnham (1947). *Modern Woman: The Lost Sex*. Universal Library.

39. L. J. Rupp (1982). The Survival of American Feminism: The Women's Movement in the Postwar Period. In R. H. Bremner and G. W. Reichard (Eds). *Reshaping America: Society and Institutions, 1945–1960* (33–65). Ohio State University Press.

40. Lundberg & Farnham, 1947.

41. Vandenberg-Daves, 2014.

42. A. Rich (1986). *Of Woman Born: Motherhood as Experience and Institution* (2nd ed.). W. W. Norton & Company.

43. R. Rapoport, R. N. Rapoport & Z. Strelitz (1977). *Fathers, Mothers, and Others: Towards New Alliances*. Routledge & Kegan Paul.

44. UNICEF UK (2019). Insert from the Baby Friendly Initiative: Infant Feeding and Relationships. *Online*.

45. S. Hays (1998). *The Cultural Contradictions of Motherhood*. Yale University Press.

46. M. Sunderland (2016). *What Every Parent Needs to Know: Love, Nurture and Play with Your Child* (2nd ed.). Dorling Kindersley.

47. R. Johnson & R. Cotmore (2015). *National Evaluation of the Graded Care Profile*. NSPCC.

48. Wirral Safeguarding Children Board (Undated). *Graded Care Profile for Wirral Children and Young People*.

49. See H. McCarthy (2020). *Double Lives: A History of Working Motherhood*. Bloomsbury. K. Swinth (2018). *Feminism's Forgotten Fight: The Unfinished Struggle for Work and Family*. Harvard University Press.

50. J. Senior (2014). *All Joy and No Fun: The Paradox of Modern Parenthood*. HarperCollins.

51. M. Doepke & F. Zilibotti (2019). *Love, Money, and Parenting: How Economics Explains the Way We Raise Our Kids*. Princeton University Press.

52. A. O'Reilly (2016). *Matricentric Feminism: Theory, Activism, Practice*. Demeter Press.

53. J. B. Wolf (2011). *Is Breast Best? Taking on the Breastfeeding Experts and the New High Stakes of Motherhood*. New York University Press.

54. R. Edwards & V. Gillies (2013). 'Where Are the Parents?': Changing Parenting Responsibilities Between the 1960s and the 2010s. In C. Faircloth, D. M. Hoffman & L. L. Layne (Eds). *Parenting in Global*

Perspective: Negotiating Ideologies of Kinship, Self and Politics (21–35). Routledge.

55. S. Menkedick (2020). *Ordinary Insanity: Fear and the Silent Crisis of Motherhood in America.* Pantheon Books.

56. C. McAteer (2023). Drinking alcohol BEFORE you're pregnant can alter your baby's face, study warns. *Netmums.*

57. X. Liu, M. Kayser, S. A. Kushner, et al. (2023). Association Between Prenatal Alcohol Exposure and Children's Facial Shape. A Prospective Population-Based Cohort Study. *Human Reproduction, 38*(5), 961–72.

58. National Center for Statistics and Analysis (2023). *Children: 2021 Data (Traffic Safety Facts. Report No. DOT HS 813 456).*

59. S. Dein (2016). The Anthropology of Uncertainty: Magic, Witchcraft and Risk and Forensic Implications. *Journal of Forensic Anthropology, 1,* 107.

60. Rich, 1986.

61. T. F. Charlton (2013). The Impossibility of the Good Black Mother. In A. N. Nathman (Ed.). *The Good Mother Myth: Redefining Motherhood to Fit Reality* (177–84). Seal Press.

62. P. H. Collins (2009). *Black Feminist Thought: Knowledge, Consciousness, and the Politics of Empowerment* (2nd ed.). Routledge.

63. S. Elliott, R. Powell & J. Brenton (2015). Being a Good Mom: Low-Income, Black Single mothers Negotiate Intensive Mothering. *Journal of Family Issues, 36*(3), 351–70.

64. P. H. Collins (1994). Shifting the Center: Race, Class, and Feminist Theorizing About Motherhood. In E. N. Glenn, G. Chang & L. R. Forcey (Eds). *Mothering: Ideology, Experience and Agency* (45–65). Routledge.

65. D. E. Roberts (1993). Racism and Patriarchy in the Meaning of Motherhood. *American University Journal of Gender, Social Policy & the Law, 1*(1), 1–38.

66. J. Randles (2021). 'Willing to Do Anything for My Kids': Inventive Mothering, Diapers, and the Inequalities of Carework. *American Sociological Review, 86*(1), 35–59.

67. J. C. Nash (2021). *Birthing Black Mothers.* Duke University Press.

68. K. L. H. Harp & A. M. Bunting (2020). The Racialized Nature of Child Welfare Policies and the Social Control of Black Bodies. *Social Politics, 27*(2), 258–81.

69. A. Frederick (2017). Risky Mothers and the Normalcy Project: Women with Disabilities Negotiate Scientific Motherhood. *Gender & Society, 31*(1), 74–95.

70. M. F. Gibson (2014). Upsetting Expertise: Disability and Queer Resistance. In M. F. Gibson (Ed.). *Queering Motherhood: Narrative and Theoretical Perspectives* (203–218). Demeter Press.

71. R. Solinger (2000). *Wake Up Little Susie: Single Pregnancy and Race Before Roe v. Wade* (2nd ed.). Routledge. Senate of Canada (2018). *The Shame is Ours: Forced Adoptions of the Babies of Unmarried Mothers in Post-war Canada.* D. Kennedy (2021, 25 May). Mothers Demand Apology Over Forced Adoptions. *BBC News.* Community Affairs References Committee (2012). *Commonwealth Contribution to Former Forced Adoption Policies and Practices.* Parliament House. N. Jones (2018, 10 May). Plea for Adoption Inquiry: 'I Tried to Photograph Her with My Eyes.' *New Zealand Herald.* M. Milotte (2021, 27 January). Forced Adoptions: An Appalling Vista? *Irish Times.*

72. Solinger, 2000.

73. Community Affairs References Committee, 2012. Senate of Canada, 2018.

74. S. Unger (Ed.) (1977). The Destruction of American Indian Families. Association on American Indian Affairs. Human Rights and Equal Opportunity Commission (1997). *Bringing Them Home: National Inquiry into the Separation of Aboriginal and Torres Strait Islander Children from Their Families.* P. Johnston (2016, 26 July). Revisiting the 'Sixties Scoop' of Indigenous Children. *Policy Options.* A. Smale (2017, 14 November). Our Stolen Generation: A Shameful Legacy. The Spinoff.

75. Human Rights and Equal Opportunity Commission, 1997.

76. Justice E. C. Kimelman (1985). *No Quiet Place: Review Committee on Indian and Metis Adoption and Placements.* Manitoba Community Services.

77. Government of Canada (2020). *Reducing the Number of Indigenous Children in Care.* Australian Government (2023). *Child Protection Australia 2020–21.* Oranga Tamariki: The Ministry for Children (2023, June). *Update on What is Happening with Entries into Care.*

78. P. Bywaters, J. Scourfield, C. Webb, et al. (2019). Paradoxical Evidence on Ethnic Inequities in Child Welfare: Towards a Research Agenda. *Children and Youth Services Review,* 96, 145–54.

79. P. Bywaters and the Child Welfare Inequalities Project Team (2020). *The Child Welfare Inequalities Project: Final Report.*

80. D. L. Bennett, D. K. Schlüter, G. Melis, et al. (2022). Child Poverty and Children Entering Care in England, 2015–20: A Longitudinal Ecological Study at the Local Area Level. *The Lancet Public Health,* 7(6), 496–503.

81. B. Featherstone, A. Gupta, K. Morris & S. White (2018). *Protecting Children: A Social Model.* Policy Press.

82. Wirral Safeguarding Children Board, undated.

83. D. Roberts (2022). *Torn Apart: How the Child Welfare System Destroys Black Families – And How Abolition Can Build a Safer World.* Basic Books.

84. L. Brown, M. Callahan, S. Strega, et al. (2009). Manufacturing Ghost Fathers: The Paradox of Father Presence and Absence in Child Welfare. *Child & Family Social Work, 14*(1), 25–34.

85. Roberts, 2022.

86. A. Bilson & P. Bywaters (2020). Born into Care: Evidence of a Failed State. *Children and Youth Services Review, 116.*

87. C. Mason, K. Broadhurst, H. Ward, et al. (2022). *Born into Care: Developing Best Practice Guidelines for When the State Intervenes at Birth.* Nuffield Family Justice Observatory.

88. R. Brown & H. Ward (2013). *Decision-Making Within a Child's Timeframe: An Overview of Current Research Evidence for Family Justice Professionals Concerning Child Development and the Impact of Maltreatment.* Childhood Wellbeing Research Centre.

89. L. Bunting, C. McCartan, J. McGhee, et al. (2018). Trends in Child Protection Across the UK: A Comparative Analysis. *British Journal of Social Work, 48*(5), 1154–75.

90. C. Mason, K. Broadhurst, H. Ward, et al., 2022.

91. Community Affairs References Committee, 2012.

92. Human Rights and Equal Opportunity Commission, 1997.

93. K. L. Nixon, H. L. Radtke & L. M. Tutty (2013). 'Every Day It Takes a Piece of You Away': Experiences of Grief and Loss Among Abused Mothers Involved with Child Protective Services. *Journal of Public Child Welfare, 7*(2), 172–93.

94. Z. Williams (2014, 26 April). Is Misused Neuroscience Defining Early Years and Child Protection Policy? *Guardian.*

95. Birthrights (2022). *Systemic Racism, Not Broken Bodies: An Inquiry into Racial Injustice and Human Rights in UK Maternity Care.*

96. E. J. Unsworth (2021). *After the Storm: Postnatal Depression and the Utter Weirdness of New Motherhood.* Profile Books.

97. K. Logan (2023). *The Unfamiliar: A Queer Motherhood Memoir.* Virago.

98. I. St James-Roberts, R. Garratt, C. Powell, et al. (2019). A Support Package for Parents of Excessively Crying Infants: Development and Feasibility Study. *Health Technol Assess, 23*(56).

99. Boots Family Trust Alliance (2013). *Perinatal Mental Health: Experiences of Women and Health Professionals.*

100. V. Harrison, D. Moore & L. Lazard (2020). Supporting Perinatal Anxiety in the Digital Age; A Qualitative Exploration of Stressors and Support Strategies. *BMC Pregnancy and Childbirth, 20,* 1–20.

101. H. Watson, D. Harrop, E. Walton, et al. (2019). A Systematic Review of Ethnic Minority Women's Experiences of Perinatal Mental Health Conditions and Services in Europe. *PLoS One, 14*(1). V. Schmied, E.

Black, N. Naidoo, et al. (2017). Migrant Women's Experiences, Meanings and Ways of Dealing with Postnatal Depression: A Meta-Ethnographic Study. *PLoS One, 12*(3).

102. A. Ahmed, D. E. Stewart, L. Teng, et al. (2008). Experiences of Immigrant New Mothers with Symptoms of Depression. *Archives of Women's Mental Health, 11,* 295–303.

103. Spock, 1946.

104. K. Manne (2019). *Down Girl: The Logic of Misogyny.* Penguin Books.

105. C. Merchant (2020). *The Death of Nature: Women, Ecology and the Scientific Revolution* (2nd ed.). HarperCollins.

106. Collins, 2009.

107. S. Mendus (1994). John Stuart Mill and Harriet Taylor on Women and Marriage. *Utilitas, 6*(2), 287–99.

108. J. S. Mill (1869). *The Subjection of Women.* Alpha Editions.

109. Quoted in McClintock, 1995.

110. S. Federici (1975). *Wages Against Housework.* Falling Wall Press.

111. J. L. Martucci (2015). *Back to the Breast: Natural Motherhood and Breastfeeding in America.* University of Chicago Press.

112. L. Scott (2020). *The Double X Economy: The Epic Potential of Empowering Women.* Faber & Faber.

113. C. Faircloth (2013). *Militant Lactivism? Attachment Parenting and Intensive Motherhood in the UK and France.* Berghahn Books.

114. B. P. Meier, A. J. Dillard & C. M. Lappas (2019). Naturally Better? A Review of the Natural-is-better Bias. *Social and Personality Psychology Compass, 13*(8).

115. R. Bellamy & S. Osaka (2020). Unnatural Climate Solutions? *Nature Climate Change, 10*(2), 98–9.

116. Traverse (2021). *Carbon Capture Usage and Storage: Public Dialogue.* Department for Business, Energy & Industrial Strategy, UKRI and Sciencewise.

117. E. Badinter (2011). *The Conflict: How Overzealous Motherhood Undermines the Status of Women.* Picador.

118. E. Biss (2015). *On Immunity: An Inoculation.* Fitzcarraldo Editions.

119. S. de Beauvoir (2015). *The Second Sex.* Translated by C. Borde & S. Malovany-Chevallier. Vintage Books.

120. L. Jordanova (1989). *Sexual Visions: Images of Gender in Science and Medicine Between the Eighteenth and Twentieth Centuries.* University of Wisconsin Press.

121. C. B. Stendler (1950). Sixty Years of Child Training Practices: Revolution in the Nursery. *The Journal of Pediatrics, 36*(1), 122–34.

122. Faircloth, 2013.

123. C. Kilroy (2023). *Soldier Sailor*. Faber & Faber.

124. P. Hamilton (2021). *Black Mothers and Attachment Parenting: A Black Feminist Analysis of Intensive Mothering in Britain and Canada*. Bristol University Press.

125. See for example R. Parker (2005). *Torn in Two: The Experience of Maternal Ambivalence* (2nd ed.). Virago.

126. V. Gillies (2013, April). From Baby Brain to Conduct Disorder: The New Determinism in the Classroom. In *Gender and Education Association Conference* (vol. 25, 82–99).

127. M. Vicedo (2013). *The Nature and Nurture of Love: From Imprinting to Attachment in Cold War America*. University of Chicago Press.

128. Quoted in *Der Spiegel* (2010, 26 August). *Spiegel* Interview with French Feminist Elisabeth Badinter: Women Aren't Chimpanzees. *Spiegel Online*.

129. S. Hustvedt (2021). *Mothers, Fathers, and Others: New Essays*. Sceptre.

130. S. Knott (2019). *Mother: An Unconventional History*. Penguin.

131. R. A. LeVine & S. LeVine (2016). *Do Parents Matter: Why Japanese Babies Sleep Soundly, Mexican Siblings Don't Fight, and American Parents Should Just Relax*. PublicAffairs.

132. I. Tattersall (2022). Foreword. In T. Pievani. *Imperfection: A Natural History* (ix-xii). MIT Press.

133. S. B. Hrdy (2011). *Mothers and Others: The Evolutionary Origins of Mutual Understanding*. Harvard University Press.

134. T. S. Weisner, R. Gallimore, M. K. Bacon, et al. (1977). My Brother's Keeper: Child and Sibling Caretaking. *Current Anthropology, 18*(2), 169–90. H. Barry III & L. M. Paxson (1971). Infancy and Early Childhood: Cross-cultural Codes 2. *Ethnology, 10*(4), 466–508.

135. D. F. Lancy (2022). *The Anthropology of Childhood: Cherubs, Chattel, Changelings* (3rd ed.). Cambridge University Press.

136. McCarthy, 2020.

137. J. Jones (2010). *Labor of Love, Labor of Sorrow: Black Women, Work, and the Family, from Slavery to the Present*. Basic Books.

138. J. Johow & E. Voland (2014). Family Among Cooperative Breeders: Challenges and Offerings to Attachment Theory from Evolutionary Anthropology. In H. Otto & H. Keller (Eds). *Different Faces of Attachment: Cultural Variations on a Universal Human Need* (27–49). Cambridge University Press.

139. Hrdy, 2011.

140. K. Hawkes (2010). How Grandmother Effects Plus Individual Variation in Frailty Shape Fertility and Mortality: Guidance from Human–Chimpanzee Comparisons. *Proceedings of the National Academy of Sciences, 107* (supplement 2), 8977–84.

141. P. N. Stearns (2015). Childhood Emotions in Modern Western History. In P. S. Fass. (Ed.). *The Routledge History of Childhood in the Western World* (158–73). Routledge.

142. Ladd-Taylor, 1994.

143. D. F. Lancy (2014). 'Babies Aren't Persons': A Survey of Delayed Personhood. In H. Otto & H. Keller (Eds). *Different Faces of Attachment: Cultural Variations of a Universal Human Need* (66–112). Cambridge University Press.

144. K. R. Bradley (2015). Images of Childhood in Classical Antiquity. In P. S. Fass (Ed.). *The Routledge History of Childhood in the Western World* (17–38). Routledge.

145. D. I. Kertzer (1993). *Sacrificed for Honor: Italian Infant Abandonment and the Politics of Reproductive Control.* Beacon Press.

146. E. Badinter (1981). *The Myth of Motherhood: An Historical View of the Maternal Instinct.* Souvenir Press (E & A).

147. V. Fildes (1988). The English Wet-Nurse and Her Role in Infant Care 1538–1800. *Medical History, 32*(2), 142–73.

148. C. Tomalin (1997). *Jane Austen: A Life.* Penguin.

149. Quoted in L. Schiebinger (1993). Why Mammals Are Called Mammals: Gender Politics in Eighteenth-century Natural History. *The American Historical Review, 98*(2), 382–411.

150. Badinter, 1981.

151. Hustvedt, 2021.

152. C. B. Canning (1935). *Ethical Aspects of Family Life.* In G. St Aubyn, (Ed.). *The Family Book: A Comprehensive Guide – Primarily for Parents* (627–61).

153. Spock, 1946.

154. P. Leach (1977). *Baby and Child: From Birth to Age Five.* Michael Joseph.

155. L. Held & A. Rutherford (2012). Can't a Mother Sing the Blues? Postpartum Depression and the Construction of Motherhood in Late 20th-century America. *History of Psychology, 15*(2), 107–23.

156. Hustvedt, 2021.

157. L. E. Sockol, C. N. Epperson & J. P. Barber (2014). The Relationship Between Maternal Attitudes and Symptoms of Depression and Anxiety Among Pregnant and Postpartum First-Time Mothers. *Archives of Women's Mental Health, 17*(3), 199–212.

158. A. Fonseca, F. Monteiro & M. C. Canavarro (2018). Dysfunctional Beliefs Towards Motherhood and Postpartum Depressive and Anxiety Symptoms: Uncovering the Role of Experiential Avoidance. *Journal of Clinical Psychology, 74*(12), 2134–44.

159. Mumsnet (2015). Experiences of Postnatal Depression: Survey Results.
160. E. K. Mollard (2014). A Qualitative Meta-Synthesis and Theory of Postpartum Depression. *Issues in Mental Health Nursing, 35*(9), 656–63.
161. C. T. Beck (2002). Postpartum Depression: A Metasynthesis. *Qualitative Health Research, 12*(4), 453–72.
162. Harrison, Moore & Lazard, 2020.
163. Mollard, 2014.
164. S. Button, A. Thornton, S. Lee, et al. (2017). Seeking Help for Perinatal Psychological Distress: A Meta-Synthesis of Women's Experiences. *British Journal of General Practice, 67*(663), 692–9.
165. C. Thomas (1997). The Baby and the Bath Water: Disabled Women and Motherhood in Social Context. *Sociology of Health & Illness, 19*(5), 622–43.
166. J. N. Daniels (2019). Disabled Mothering? Outlawed, Overlooked and Severely Prohibited: Interrogating Ableism in Motherhood. *Social Inclusion, 7*(1), 114–23.
167. A. Windsor (2014). An Existential Crisis Is Born. In A. N. Nathman (Ed.). *The Good Mother Myth: Redefining Motherhood to Fit Reality* (121–8). Seal Press.
168. Hamilton, 2021.
169. Rich, 1986.

2. Why Science Can't Talk

1. UCI (2016, 5 January). Put the Cellphone Away! Fragmented Baby Care Can Affect Brain Development. *UCI News*.
2. J. Molet, K. Heins, X. Zhuo, et al. (2016). Fragmentation and High Entropy of Neonatal Experience Predict Adolescent Emotional Outcome. *Translational Psychiatry, 6*.
3. P. Sumner, S. Vivian-Griffiths, J. Boivin, et al. (2014). The Association Between Exaggeration in Health Related Science News and Academic Press Releases: Retrospective Observational Study. *BMJ, 349*.
4. J. Schat, F. G. Bossema, M. E. Numans, et al. (2018). Exaggerated Health News: Association Between Exaggeration in University Press Releases and Exaggeration in News Media Coverage. *Nederlands Tijdschrift Voor Geneeskunde, 162*(1).
5. A. Park (2016, 6 January). Cell-Phone Distracted Parenting Can Have Long-Term Consequences: Study. *Time*.
6. D. Kahneman (2011). *Thinking, Fast and Slow*. Penguin.
7. T. Vigen (2015). *Spurious Correlations: Correlation Does Not Equal Causation*. Hachette Books.

8. Quoted in D. V. M. Bishop (2020). The Psychology of Experimental Psychologists: Overcoming Cognitive Constraints to Improve Research: The 47th Sir Frederic Bartlett Lecture. *Quarterly Journal of Experimental Psychology, 73*(1), 1–19.

9. J. R. Harris (2009). *The Nurture Assumption: Why Children Turn Out the Way They Do* (2nd ed.). Simon & Schuster.

10. J. P. Simmons, L. D. Nelson & U. Simonsohn (2011). False-Positive Psychology: Undisclosed Flexibility in Data Collection and Analysis Allows Presenting Anything as Significant. *Psychological Science, 22*(11), 1359–66.

11. R. L. Wasserstein & N. A. Nicole (2016). The ASA's Statement on p-Values: Context, Process, and Purpose. *The American Statistician, 70*(2), 129–33.

12. C. M. Bennett, A. A. Baird, M. B. Miller & G. L. Wolford (2009). Neural Correlates of Interspecies Perspective Taking in the Post-Mortem Atlantic Salmon: An Argument for Multiple Comparisons Correction. *Neuroimage, 47* (suppl. 1), S125.

13. N. Silver (2012). *The Signal and the Noise: The Art and Science of Prediction*. Penguin.

14. D. P. Vivekananthan, M. S. Penn, S. K. Sapp, et al. (2003). Use of Antioxidant Vitamins for the Prevention of Cardiovascular Disease: Meta-Analysis of Randomised Trials. *The Lancet, 361*(9374), 2017–23.

15. L. S. Pagani & C. Fitzpatrick (2018). Children's Early Disruptive Behavior Predicts Later Coercive Behavior and Binge Drinking by Mothers. *Journal of Pediatric Nursing: Nursing Care of Children and Families, 39*, 15–20.

16. Bishop, 2020.

17. T. S. Kuhn (1970). *The Structure of Scientific Revolutions* (2nd ed.). University of Chicago Press.

18. Quoted in G. Tett (2021). *Anthro-Vision: How Anthropology Can Explain Business and Life*. Penguin.

19. S. Harding (2008). *Sciences from Below: Feminisms, Postcolonialities, and Modernities*. Duke University Press.

20. H. E. Longino (1990). *Science as Social Knowledge: Values and Objectivity in Scientific Inquiry*. Princeton University Press.

21. M. Weisberger (2023, 30 June). Shattering the Myth of Men as Hunters and Women as Gatherers. *CNN*.

22. A. Anderson, S. Chilczuk, K. Nelson, et al. (2023). The Myth of Man the Hunter: Women's Contribution to the Hunt Across Ethnographic Contexts. *PLoS One, 18*(6).

23. A. McClintock (1995). *Imperial Leather: Race, Gender, and Sexuality in the Colonial Contest*. Routledge.

24. C. Smith-Rosenberg & C. Rosenberg (1973). The Female Animal: Medical and Biological Views of Woman and Her Role in Nineteenth-Century America. *The Journal of American History*, 60(2), 332–56.

25. J. Lewis (1984). *Women in England, 1870–1950: Sexual Divisions and Social Change*. Wheatsheaf Books.

26. H. Maudsley (1874). Sex in Mind and in Education. *Popular Science Monthly*, 5.

27. Lewis, 1984.

28. Smith-Rosenberg & Rosenberg, 1973.

29. C. E. Russett (1989). *Sexual Science: The Victorian Construction of Womanhood*. Harvard University Press.

30. Lewis, 1984.

31. Smith-Rosenberg & Rosenberg, 1973.

32. Ipsos (2023). *Ipsos Veracity Index 2023: Trust in Professions Survey*.

33. Ipsos (2023). *Ipsos Global Trustworthiness Index: Who Does the World Trust?*

34. D. E. Eyer (1992). *Mother-Infant Bonding: A Scientific Fiction*. Yale University Press.

35. C. Faircloth (2010). 'What Science Says Is Best': Parenting Practices, Scientific Authority and Maternal Identity. *Sociological Research Online*, 15(4), 85–98.

36. B. S. Bradley (1989). *Visions of Infancy: A Critical Introduction to Child Psychology*. Polity Press.

37. M. H. Klaus & J. H. Kennell (1976). *Maternal-Infant Bonding: The Impact of Early Separation or Loss on Family Development*. The C. V. Mosby Company.

38. A. Loader, on behalf of the National Childbirth Trust (1980). *Pregnancy & Parenthood*. Oxford University Press.

39. M. E. Lamb (1982). Early Contact and Maternal-Infant Bonding: One Decade Later. *Pediatrics*, 70(5), 763–8. M. Herbert, W. Sluckin & A. Sluckin (1982). Mother-To-Infant 'Bonding'. *Journal of Child Psychology and Psychiatry*, 23(3), 205–21.

40. J. E. Brody (1983, 29 March). Influential Theory on 'Bonding' at Birth Is Now Questioned. *New York Times*.

41. J. H. Kennell & M. H. Klaus (1984). Mother-Infant Bonding: Weighing the Evidence. *Developmental Review*, 4(3), 275–82.

42. A. Tversky & D. Kahneman (1971). Belief in the Law of Small Numbers. *Psychological Bulletin*, 76(2), 105–10.

43. Kahneman, 2011.

44. Quoted in D. Spiegelhalter (2019). *The Art of Statistics: Learning from Data*. Pelican.

45. I. Plewis (Ed.) (2007). *The Millennium Cohort Study: Technical Report on Sampling* (4th ed.). Centre for Longitudinal Studies.

46. J. Henrich, S. Heine & A. Norenzayan (2010). The Weirdest People in the World? *Behavioral and Brain Sciences, 33*(2–3), 61–135.

47. Open Science Collaboration (2015). Estimating the Reproducibility of Psychological Science. *Science, 349*(6251).

48. J. Dryden (2012, 30 January). *Mom's Love Good for Child's Brain.* Washington University in St Louis.

49. J. L. Luby, D. M. Barch, A. Belden, et al. (2012). Maternal Support in Early Childhood Predicts Larger Hippocampal Volumes at School Age. *Proceedings of the National Academy of Sciences, 109*(8), 2854–9.

50. K. G. Noble, S. M. Houston, N. H. Brito, et al. (2015). Family Income, Parental Education and Brain Structure in Children and Adolescents. *Nature Neuroscience, 18*(5), 773–8.

51. J. L. Luby, A. Belden, M. P. Harms, et al. (2016). Preschool is a Sensitive Period for the Influence of Maternal Support on the Trajectory of Hippocampal Development. *Proceedings of the National Academy of Sciences, 113*(20), 5742–7.

52. J. Dryden (2016, 25 April). *Nurturing During Preschool Years Boosts Child's Brain Growth.* Washington University School of Medicine.

53. F. MacRae (2016, 27 April). Why a Mother's Love Really Does Matter: Nurturing Helps Children's Brains Grow at TWICE the Rate of Those Who Are 'Neglected'. *Daily Mail.*

54. D. S. Weisberg, F. C. Keil, J. Goodstein, et al. (2008). The Seductive Allure of Neuroscience Explanations. *Journal of Cognitive Neuroscience, 20*(3), 470–7.

55. D. S. Weisberg, J. C. Taylor & E. J. Hopkins (2015). Deconstructing the Seductive Allure of Neuroscience Explanations. *Judgment and Decision Making, 10*(5), 429–41.

56. D. Fernandez-Duque, J. Evans, C. Christian & S. D. Hodges (2015). Superfluous Neuroscience Information Makes Explanations of Psychological Phenomena More Appealing. *Journal of Cognitive Neuroscience, 27*(5), 926–44.

57. J. T. Bruer (1999). *The Myth of the First Three Years: A New Understanding of Early Brain Development and Lifelong Learning.* Simon and Schuster.

58. The studies showing this are summarised in S. J. Blakemore (2018). *Inventing Ourselves: The Secret Life of the Teenage Brain.* Doubleday.

59. J. Kagan (1998). *Three Seductive Ideas.* Harvard University Press.

60. J. P. Shonkoff & S. N. Bales (2011). Science Does Not Speak for Itself: Translating Child Development Research for the Public and its Policymakers. *Child Development, 82*(1), 17–32.

61. National Scientific Council on the Developing Child (2007). *The Science of Early Childhood Development: Closing the Gap Between What We Know and What We Do.* Center on the Developing Child, Harvard University.

62. R. Tallis (2011) *Aping Mankind: Neuromania, Darwinitis and the Misrepresentation of Humanity.* Acumen.

63. Kagan, 1998.

64. Center on the Developing Child at Harvard University (2007). *A Science -Based Framework for Early Childhood Policy: Using Evidence to Improve Outcomes in Learning, Behavior, and Health for Vulnerable Children.*

65. P. Levitt (2003). Structural and Functional Maturation of the Developing Primate Brain. *Journal of Pediatrics, 143*(4), 35–45. C. S. Monk, S. J. Webb & C. A. Nelson (2001). Prenatal Neurobiological Development: Molecular Mechanisms and Anatomical Change. *Developmental Neuropsychology, 19*(2), 211–36.

66. S. J. Webb, C. S. Monk & C. A. Nelson (2001). Mechanisms of Postnatal Neurobiological Development: Implications for Human Development. *Developmental Neuropsychology, 19*(2), 147–71.

67. P. A. Howard-Jones (2014). Neuroscience and Education: Myths and Messages. *Nature Reviews Neuroscience, 15*(12), 817–24.

68. M. Cobb (2020). *The Idea of the Brain: A History.* Profile Books.

69. Howard-Jones, 2014.

70. National Scientific Council on the Developing Child (2014). *Excessive Stress Disrupts the Architecture of the Developing Brain: Working Paper 3.*

71. M. M. Loman & M. R. Gunnar (2010). Early Experience and the Development of Stress Reactivity and Regulation in Children. *Neuroscience & Biobehavioral Reviews, 34*(6), 867–76.

72. K. Bernard, A. Frost, C. B. Bennett & O. Lindhiem (2017). Maltreatment and Diurnal Cortisol Regulation: A Meta-Analysis. *Psychoneuroendocrinology, 78,* 57–67.

73. S. Schär, I. Mürner-Lavanchy, S. J. Schmidt, et al. (2022). Child Maltreatment and Hypothalamic-Pituitary-Adrenal Axis Functioning: A Systematic Review and Meta-Analysis. *Frontiers in Neuroendocrinology, 66.*

74. D. M. Lyons & K. J. Parker (2007). Stress Inoculation-Induced Indications of Resilience in Monkeys. *Journal of Traumatic Stress, 20*(4), 423–33.

75. K. Gapp, S. Soldado-Magraner, M. Alvarez-Sánchez, et al. (2014). Early Life Stress in Fathers Improves Behavioural Flexibility in Their Offspring. *Nature Communications, 5*(1), 5466.

76. See for example S. Moullin, J. Waldfogel & E. Washbrook (2014). *Baby Bonds: Parenting, Attachment and a Secure Base for Children.* Sutton Trust.

77. D. F. Narvaez (2011, 11 December). Dangers of 'Crying It Out'. *Psychology Today.*

78. T. M. Pollard & G. H. Ice (2007). Measuring Hormonal Variation in the Hypothalamic Pituitary Adrenal Axis: Cortisol. In G. H. Ice & G. D. James (Eds). *Measuring Stress in Humans: A Practical Guide for the Field* (122–57). Cambridge University Press.

79. Ibid.

80. A. S. Karlamangla, E. M. Friedman, T. E. Seeman, et al. (2013). Daytime Trajectories of Cortisol: Demographic and Socioeconomic Differences – Findings from the National Study of Daily Experiences. *Psychoneuroendocrinology, 38*(11), 2585–97.

81. O. James (2010). *How Not to F*** Them Up.* Vermilion.

82. W. Middlemiss, D. A. Granger, W. A. Goldberg & L. Nathans (2012). Asynchrony of Mother–Infant Hypothalamic–Pituitary–Adrenal Axis Activity Following Extinction of Infant Crying Responses Induced During the Transition to Sleep. *Early Human Development, 88*(4), 227–32.

83. G. Timothy (2018). *Mum Face: The Memoir of a Woman Who Gained Her Baby and Lost Her Shit.* HarperCollins.

84. See for example H. Ball & P. S. Blair (2021). *The Health Professional's Guide to: 'Caring for Your Baby at Night'.* UNICEF UK. V. Gillies, R. Edwards & N. Horsley (2017). *Challenging the Politics of Early Intervention: Who's 'Saving' Children and Why.* Policy Press.

85. A. N. Schore (1994). *Affect Regulation and the Origin of the Self: The Neurobiology of Emotional Development.* Erlbaum.

86. S. Gerhardt (2004). *Why Love Matters: How Affection Shapes a Baby's Brain.* Routledge.

87. I. Branchi, J. P. Curley, I. D'Andrea, et al. (2013). Early Interactions with Mother and Peers Independently Build Adult Social Skills and Shape BDNF and Oxytocin Receptor Brain Levels. *Psychoneuroendocrinology, 38*(4), 522–32. P. Y. Lin & K. P. Su (2007). A Meta-Analytic Review of Double-Blind, Placebo-Controlled Trials of Antidepressant Efficacy of Omega-3 Fatty Acids. *Journal of Clinical Psychiatry, 68*(7), 1056–61. S. Gerhardt (2014). *Why Love Matters: How Affection Shapes a Baby's Brain* (2nd ed.). Routledge.

88. H. Rose & S. Rose (2016). *Can Neuroscience Change our Minds?* John Wiley & Sons.

89. A. Palmer (2012, 28 October). These Two Brains Belong to Three Year Olds, So Why is One So Much Bigger? *Daily Telegraph.*

90. G. Allen & I. Duncan Smith (2008). *Early Intervention: Good Parents, Great Kids, Better Citizens.* The Centre for Social Justice and the Smith Institute.

91. G. Allen (2011). *Early Intervention: The Next Steps.* HM Government.

92. G. Allen (2011). *Early Intervention: Smart Investment, Massive Savings.* HM Government.

93. D. Wastell & S. White (2012). Blinded by Neuroscience: Social Policy, the Family and the Infant Brain. *Families, Relationships and Societies,* *1*(3), 397–414.

94. B. D. Perry (2002). Childhood Experience and the Expression of Genetic Potential: What Childhood Neglect Tells Us About Nature and Nurture. *Brain and Mind,* *3*(1), 79–100.

95. Gillies, Edwards & Horsley, 2017.

96. Rose & Rose, 2016.

97. P. Lewis & S. Boseley (2010, 9 April). Iain Duncan Smith 'Distorted' Research on Childhood Neglect and Brain Size. *Guardian.*

98. R. Gilbert, C. S. Widom, K. Browne, et al. (2009). Burden and Consequences of Child Maltreatment in High-Income Countries. *The Lancet,* *373*(9657), 68–81.

99. M. I. Gerin, E. Hanson, E. Viding & E. J. McCrory (2019). A Review of Childhood Maltreatment, Latent Vulnerability and the Brain: Implications for Clinical Practice and Prevention. *Adoption & Fostering,* *43*(3), 310–28.

100. J. Macvarish (2016). *Neuroparenting: The Expert Invasion of Family Life.* Palgrave Macmillan.

101. Save the Children (2016). *Lighting up Young Brains: How Parents, Carers and Nurseries Support Children's Brain Development in the First Five Years.*

102. G. Allen (2011). *Early Intervention: The Next Steps.* HM Government.

103. Rose & Rose, 2016.

104. HM Government (2021). *The Best Start for Life: A Vision for the 1001 Critical Days. The Early Years Healthy Development Review Report.*

105. Parent-Infant Foundation (2024). First 1001 Days Movement: Members. *Online.*

106. zerotothree.org.

107. Blakemore, 2018.

108. A. Dickerson & G. K. Popli (2016). Persistent Poverty and Children's Cognitive Development: Evidence from the UK Millennium Cohort Study. *Journal of the Royal Statistical Society: Series A (Statistics in Society),* *179*(2), 535–58.

109. E. T. Lai, S. Wickham, C. Law, et al. (2019). Poverty Dynamics and Health in Late Childhood in the UK: Evidence from the Millennium Cohort Study. *Archives of Disease in Childhood,* *104*, 1049–55.

110. National Academies of Sciences, Engineering, and Medicine (2019). *A Roadmap to Reducing Child Poverty*. National Academies Press.

111. Eyer, 1992.

112. K. Thomas (1973). *Religion and the Decline of Magic: Studies in Popular Beliefs in Sixteenth and Seventeenth-Century England*. Penguin Books.

113. C. Nemeroff & P. Rozin (2000). The Makings of the Magical Mind: The Nature and Function of Sympathetic Magical Thinking. In K. Rosengren, C. Johnson & P. Harris (Eds). *Imagining the Impossible: Magical, Scientific, and Religious Thinking in Children* (1–34). Cambridge University Press.

114. UCI, 2016.

115. J. Brooks-Gunn (2003). Do You Believe in Magic? What We Can Expect from Early Childhood Intervention Programs. *Social Policy Report, 17*(1).

116. Blakemore, 2018.

117. E. Zigler (2003). Forty Years of Believing in Magic is Enough. *Social Policy Report, 17*(1).

118. G. C. Sharp, L. Schellhas, S. S. Richardson & D. A. Lawlor (2019). Time to Cut the Cord: Recognizing and Addressing the Imbalance of DOHaD Research Towards the Study of Maternal Pregnancy Exposures. *Journal of Developmental Origins of Health and Disease, 10*(5), 509–12.

119. S. S. Richardson (2021). *The Maternal Imprint: The Contested Science of Maternal-Fetal Effects*. The University of Chicago Press.

120. A. D. Lyerly, L. M. Mitchell, E. M. Armstrong, et al. (2009). Risk and the Pregnant Body. *Hastings Center Report, 39*(6), 34–42.

121. Cobb, 2020.

122. K. Millett (1977). *Sexual Politics*. Virago.

3. Birthing Pains

1. T. McIntosh (2012). *A Social History of Maternity and Childbirth: Key Themes in Maternity Care*. Routledge.

2. L. Jordanova (1989). *Sexual Visions: Images of Gender in Science and Medicine Between the Eighteenth and Twentieth Centuries*. University of Wisconsin Press.

3. T. Cosslett (1994). *Women Writing Childbirth: Modern Discourses of Motherhood*. Manchester University Press.

4. S. Kitzinger (2006). *Birth Crisis*. Routledge.

5. P. A. Michaels (2014). *Lamaze: An International History*. Oxford University Press.

6. S. Kitzinger (2012). *Birth & Sex: The Power and the Passion.* Pinter & Martin.

7. R. Davis-Floyd & E. Davis (1996). Intuition as Authoritative Knowledge in Midwifery and Homebirth. *Medical Anthropology Quarterly, 10*(2), 237–69.

8. H. P. Dietz (2017). Women and Babies Need Protection from the Dangers of Normal Birth Ideology. *BJOG 124*(9), 1384.

9. S. Miller, E. Abalos, M. Chamillard, et al. (2016). Beyond Too Little, Too Late and Too Much, Too Soon: A Pathway Towards Evidence-Based, Respectful Maternity Care Worldwide. *The Lancet, 388*(10056), 2176–92.

10. T. Boerma, C. Ronsmans, D. Y. Melesse, et al. (2018). Global Epidemiology of Use of and Disparities in Caesarean Sections. *The Lancet, 392*(10155), 1341–8.

11. World Health Organization (2023). Trends in Maternal Mortality 2000 to 2020: Estimates by WHO, UNICEF, UNFPA, World Bank Group and UNDESA/Population Division.

12. L. Say, D. Chou, A. Gemmill, et al. (2014). Global Causes of Maternal Death: A WHO Systematic Analysis. *The Lancet Global Health, 2*(6), 323–33.

13. E. Kukura (2018). Obstetric Violence. *The Georgetown Law Journal 106*(3), 721–801.

14. J. B. Litoff (1978). *American Midwives: 1860 to the Present.* Greenwood Press.

15. S. C. Clarke, J. A. Martin & S. M. Taffel (1997). Trends and Characteristics of Births Attended by Midwives. *Statistical Bulletin (Metropolitan Life Insurance Company: 1984), 78*(1), 9–18.

16. J. H. Wolf (2009). *Deliver Me from Pain: Anesthesia and Birth in America.* The Johns Hopkins University Press.

17. J. W. Leavitt (1988). Joseph B. DeLee and the Practice of Preventive Obstetrics. *AJPH 78*(10), 1353–60.

18. J. B. DeLee (1916). Progress Toward Ideal Obstetrics. *The American Journal of Obstetrics and Diseases of Women and Children (1869–1919), 73*(3), 407.

19. Wolf, 2009.

20. Kitzinger, 2006.

21. C. Clesse, J. Lighezzolo-Alnot, S. De Lavergne, et al. (2019). Socio-Historical Evolution of the Episiotomy Practice: A Literature Review. *Women & Health, 59*(7), 760–74.

22. Michaels, 2014.

23. For the most recent data see J. A. Martin, B. E. Hamilton & M. J. Osterman (2023). Births in the United States, 2022. *NCHS Data Brief,*

477. For historical data, see this paper's appendix: A. P. Betran, J. Ye, A -B. Moller, et al. (2021). Trends and Projections of Caesarean Section Rates: Global and Regional Estimates. *BMJ Global Health*, 6(6).

24. S. C. Curtin & M. M. Park (1999). Trends in the Attendant, Place, and Timing of Births, and in the Use of Obstetric Interventions: United States, 1989–97. *National Vital Statistics Reports*, 47(27).

25. Z. Alfirevic, G. M. L. Gyte, A. Cuthbert & D. Devane (2017). Continuous Cardiotocography (CTG) as a Form of Electronic Fetal Monitoring (EFM) for Fetal Assessment During Labour. *Cochrane Database of Systematic Reviews*, (2).

26. L. M. Roth (2021). *The Business of Birth: Malpractice and Maternity Care in the United States*. New York University Press.

27. B. Hunter (2012). Midwifery, 1920–2000: The Reshaping of a Profession. In A. Borsay & B. Hunter (Eds). *Nursing and Midwifery in Britain since 1700* (151–74). Bloomsbury Publishing. McIntosh, 2012.

28. Clesse et al., 2019.

29. Hunter, 2012.

30. Maternity Care Working Party (2007). *Making Normal Birth a Reality*. RCM, RCOG, NCT.

31. G. Dick-Read (1959). *Childbirth Without Fear: The Principles and Practice of Natural Childbirth*. Pinter & Martin.

32. P. Kerley (2016, 4 May). NCT: The National Childbirth Trust's 60 Years of Advice. *BBC News Magazine*.

33. Michaels, 2014.

34. J. Kitzinger (1990). Strategies of the Early Childbirth Movement: A Case -Study of the National Childbirth Trust. In J. Garcia, R. Kilpatrick & M. Richards. *The Politics of Maternity Care: Services for Childbearing Women in Twentieth-Century Britain* (92–115). Oxford University Press.

35. C. Malacrida & T. Boulton (2014). The Best Laid Plans? Women's Choices, Expectations and Experiences in Childbirth. *Health, 18*(1), 41–59.

36. V. Harrison, D. Moore & L. Lazard (2020). Supporting Perinatal Anxiety in the Digital Age; A Qualitative Exploration of Stressors and Support Strategies. *BMC Pregnancy and Childbirth*, 20, 1–20.

37. Montgomery v Lanarkshire Health Board (2015). SC 11 [2015] 1 AC 1430.

38. D. Ockenden (2022). *Ockenden Report – Final*. HC 1219.

39. R. Reed, R. Sharman & C. Inglis (2017). Women's Descriptions of Childbirth Trauma Relating to Care Provider Actions and Interactions. *BMC Pregnancy and Childbirth*, 17, 1–10.

40. Kukura, 2018.
41. Birthrights (2013). *Dignity in Childbirth – the Dignity Survey 2013: Women's and Midwives' Experiences of UK Maternity Care.*
42. G. Moncrieff, G. M. L. Gyte, H. G. Dahlen, et al. (2022). Routine Vaginal Examinations Compared to Other Methods for Assessing Progress of Labour to Improve Outcomes for Women and Babies at Term. *Cochrane Database of Systematic Reviews*, (3).
43. Reed, Sharman & Inglis, 2017.
44. E. J. Unsworth (2021). *After the Storm: Postnatal Depression and the Utter Weirdness of New Motherhood.* Profile Books.
45. E. R. Declercq, C. Sakala, M. P. Corry, et al. (2013). *Listening to Mothers III: Pregnancy and Birth.* Childbirth Connection.
46. M. A. Bohren, H. Mehrtash, B. Fawole, et al. (2019). How Women are Treated During Facility-Based Childbirth in Four Countries: A Cross-Sectional Study with Labour Observations and Community-Based Surveys. *The Lancet, 394*, 1750–63.
47. S. Vedam, K. Stoll, T. K. Taiwo, et al. (2019). The Giving Voice to Mothers Study: Inequity and Mistreatment During Pregnancy and Childbirth in the United States. *Reproductive Health, 16*, 1–18.
48. D. L. Hoyert (2023). Maternal Mortality Rates in the United States, 2021. *NCHS Health E-Stats.*
49. M. Knight, K. Bunch, A. Felker, et al. (2023). *Saving Lives, Improving Mothers' Care: Lessons Learned to Inform Maternity Care from the UK and Ireland Confidential Enquiries into Maternal Deaths and Morbidity 2019–21.* National Perinatal Epidemiology Unit, University of Oxford.
50. S. Williams (2022, 5 April). How Serena Williams Saved Her Own Life. *Elle.*
51. K. M. Hoffman, S. Trawalter, J. R. Axt & M. N. Oliver (2016). Racial Bias in Pain Assessment and Treatment Recommendations, and False Beliefs About Biological Differences Between Blacks and Whites. *Proceedings of the National Academy of Sciences, 113*(16), 4296–301.
52. Birthrights (2022). *Systemic Racism, Not Broken Bodies: An Inquiry into Racial Injustice and Human Rights in UK Maternity Care.*
53. C. Brathwaite (2020). *I Am Not Your Baby Mother: What It's Like to Be a Black British Mother.* Quercus.
54. World Health Organization (2014). *The Prevention and Elimination of Disrespect and Abuse During Facility-Based Childbirth.*
55. C. R. Williams, C. Jerez, K. Klein, et al. (2018). Obstetric Violence: A Latin American Legal Response to Mistreatment During Childbirth. *BJOG, 125*(10), 1208–11.

56. R. Jewkes & L. Penn-Kekana (2015). Mistreatment of Women in Childbirth: Time for Action on this Important Dimension of Violence Against Women. *PLoS Medicine,* *12*(6).

57. D. A. Davis (2019). Obstetric Racism: The Racial Politics of Pregnancy, Labor, and Birthing. *Medical Anthropology,* *38*(7), 560–73.

58. R. Chadwick (2021). Breaking the Frame: Obstetric Violence and Epistemic Rupture. *Agenda,* *35*(3), 104–15.

59. A. Dawes, G. Beard, C. Pistone, et al. (2022). *Birth Injuries: The Hidden Epidemic.* Australasian Birth Trauma Association, Birth Trauma Association and Make Birth Better.

60. H. Priddis, V. Schmied & H. Dahlen (2014). Women's Experiences Following Severe Perineal Trauma: A Qualitative Study. *BMC Women's Health,* *14*, 1–11.

61. C. Criado Perez (2019). *Invisible Women: Exposing Data Bias in a World Designed for Men.* Chatto & Windus.

62. Mumsnet (2018). We Should Not be Normalising Postnatal Pain. *Online.*

63. S. Dekel, C. Stuebe & G. Dishy (2017). Childbirth Induced Posttraumatic Stress Syndrome: A Systematic Review of Prevalence and Risk Factors. *Frontiers in Psychology,* *8*, 1–10. P. D. Yildiz, S. Ayers & L. Phillips (2017). The Prevalence of Posttraumatic Stress Disorder in Pregnancy and After Birth: A Systematic Review and Meta-Analysis. *Journal of Affective Disorders,* *208*, 634–45.

64. National Institute of Mental Health (2024). Post-Traumatic Stress Disorder. *Online.*

65. C. T. Beck (2016). Posttraumatic Stress Disorder After Birth: A Metaphor Analysis. *MCN: The American Journal of Maternal/Child Nursing,* *41*(2), 76–83.

66. P. Dikmen-Yildiz, S. Ayers & L. Phillips (2018). Longitudinal Trajectories of Post-Traumatic Stress Disorder (PTSD) After Birth and Associated Risk Factors. *Journal of Affective Disorders,* *229*, 377–85.

67. K. Thomas (2020). *Birth Trauma: A Guide for You, Your Friends and Family to Coping with Post-Traumatic Stress Disorder Following Birth* (2nd ed.). Nell James Publishers.

68. S. Ayers & E. Ford (2014). Post-Traumatic Stress During Pregnancy and the Postpartum Period. In *The Oxford Handbook of Perinatal Psychology* (182–200). Oxford University Press.

69. S. Ayers, R. Bond, S. Bertullies & K. Wijma (2016). The Aetiology of Post-Traumatic Stress Following Childbirth: A Meta-Analysis and Theoretical Framework. *Psychological Medicine,* *46*, 1121–34. Dekel, Stuebe & Dishy, 2017.

70. Dawes, Beard, Pistone, et al., 2022.
71. Thomas, 2020.
72. Interview with Yania Escobar in A. Apfel (2016). *Birth Work as Care Work: Stories from Activist Birth Communities*. Kairos.
73. Birthrights (2018). *Maternal Request Caesarean*.
74. Interview with Kelly Gray in Apfel, 2016.
75. Kitzinger, 2012.
76. W. R. Trevathan (1987). *Human Birth: An Evolutionary Perspective*. Aldine de Gruyter.
77. J. K. Gupta, A. Sood, G. J. Hofmeyr & J. P. Vogel (2017). Position in the Second Stage of Labour for Women Without Epidural Anaesthesia. *Cochrane Database of Systematic Reviews*, (5).
78. T. Morris & K. McInerney (2010). Media Representations of Pregnancy and Childbirth: An Analysis of Reality Television Programs in the United States. *Birth*, 37(2), 134–40.
79. S. De Benedictis, C. Johnson, J. Roberts & H. Spiby (2019). Quantitative Insights into Televised Birth: A Content Analysis of *One Born Every Minute*. *Critical Studies in Media Communication*, 36(1), 1–17.
80. S. Robson (2022, 31 March). Parent Charity NCT Deletes Natural Birth Guidance that Says 'Mothers Will be More Satisfied'. *The i.*
81. E. Glaser (2021) *Motherhood: Feminism's Unfinished Business*. 4th Estate.
82. R. Holman (2021, 7 April). The Pros and Cons of Doing NCT. *Grazia*.
83. S. Muse, E. Dawes Gay, A. D. Aina, et al. (2018). *Setting the Standard for Holistic Care of and for Black Women*. Black Mamas Matter Alliance.
84. LGBT Foundation (2022). *Trans + Non-Binary Experiences of Maternity Services*.
85. National Institute for Health and Care Excellence (2014). *Intrapartum Care for Healthy Women and Babies. Clinical Guideline [CG190]*.
86. B. Kirkup (2015). *The Report of the Morecambe Bay Investigation*. University Hospitals of Morecambe Bay NHS Foundation Trust.
87. NHS Resolution (2023). *Annual Report and Accounts 2022/23*.
88. Birthrights, 2022.
89. World Health Organization, 2023.
90. M. D. Gunja, E. D. Gumas & R. D. Williams II (2023). *US Health Care from a Global Perspective, 2022: Accelerating Spending, Worsening Outcomes*. Commonwealth Fund.
91. K. Kennedy-Moulton, S. Miller, P. Persson, et al. (2022). *Maternal and Infant Health Inequality: New Evidence from Linked Administrative Data*. National Bureau of Economic Research.
92. Muse, Dawes Gay & Aina, et al. 2018.

93. Clarke, Martin & Taffel, 1997. J. Farb (2023). Midwives: Information on Births, Workforce, and Midwifery Education. *US Government Accountability Office, GAO-23-105861.*

94. Farb, 2023.

95. Roth, 2021.

96. J. Sandall, C. Fernandez Turienzo, D. Devane, et al. (2024). Midwife Continuity of Care Models Versus Other Models of Care for Childbearing Women. *Cochrane Database of Systematic Reviews*, (4).

97. C. S. E. Homer, N. Leap, N. Edwards & J. Sandall (2017). Midwifery Continuity of Care in an Area of High Socio-Economic Disadvantage in London: A Retrospective Analysis of Albany Midwifery Practice Outcomes Using Routine Data (1997–2009). *Midwifery*, *48*, 1–10. R. Hadebe, P. T. Seed, D. Essien, et al. (2021). Can Birth Outcome Inequality be Reduced Using Targeted Caseload Midwifery in a Deprived Diverse Inner City Population? A Retrospective Cohort Study, London, UK. *BMJ Open*, *11*(11). L. Dubay, I. Hill, B. Garrett, et al. (2020). Improving Birth Outcomes and Lowering Costs for Women on Medicaid: Impacts of 'Strong Start for Mothers and Newborns'. *Health Affairs*, *39*(6), 1042–50.

98. World Health Organization (2022). *WHO Recommendations for Care of the Preterm or Low Birthweight Infant.*

99. V. Perrotte, A. Chaudhary & A. Goodman (2020). 'At Least Your Baby Is Healthy' Obstetric Violence or Disrespect and Abuse in Childbirth Occurrence Worldwide: A Literature Review. *Open Journal of Obstetrics and Gynecology*, *10*(11), 1544–62.

100. R. Chadwick (2021). The Dangers of Minimizing Obstetric Violence. *Violence Against Women*, *29*(9), 1899–1908.

101. P. Slade, K. Balling, K. Sheen, et al. (2020). Work-Related Post-Traumatic Stress Symptoms in Obstetricians and Gynaecologists: Findings from INDIGO, a Mixed-Methods Study with a Cross-Sectional Survey and In-Depth Interviews. *BJOG*, *127*(5), 600–8.

102. C. T. Beck & R. K. Gable (2012). A Mixed Methods Study of Secondary Traumatic Stress in Labor and Delivery Nurses. *JOGNN*, *41*(6), 747–60.

103. National Institute for Health and Care Excellence (2021). *Postnatal Care [J] Perineal pain NICE Guideline NG194: Evidence Review Underpinning Recommendations.*

104. Knight, Bunch, Felker, et al., 2023. K. Chin, A. Wendt, I. M. Bennett & A. Bhat (2022). Suicide and Maternal Mortality. *Current Psychiatry Reports*, *24*(4), 239–75.

4. Feeding Frenzy

1. H. Heardman (1970). *A Way to Natural Childbirth* (2nd ed.). E&S Livingstone.

2. UNICEF (2018). *Breastfeeding: A Mother's Gift for Every Child.*

3. G. Thomson, K. Ebisch-Burton & R. Flacking (2014). Shame If You Do – Shame If You Don't: Women's Experiences of Infant Feeding. *Maternal & Child Nutrition*, 11(1), 33–46.

4. G. Palmer (2009). *The Politics of Breastfeeding: When Breasts are Bad for Business* (3rd ed.). Pinter & Martin.

5. J. C. Nash (2021). *Birthing Black Mothers*. Duke University Press.

6. B. Åström (2015). A Narrative of Fear: Advice to Mothers. *Literature and Medicine*, 33(1), 113–31.

7. A. Combe & J. Clark (1860). *The Management of Infancy: Physiological and Moral*. Kessinger Legacy Reprints.

8. E. Pritchard (1921). *The Infant: Nutrition and Management* (2nd ed.). Edward Arnold.

9. First Steps Nutrition Trust (2020). *Infant Milks in the UK: A Practical Guide for Health Professionals.*

10. J. C. Wilson & B. Andrassy (2022). Breastfeeding Experiences of Autistic Women. *MCN: The American Journal of Maternal/Child Nursing*, 47(1), 19–24.

11. D. F. Lancy (2014). 'Babies Aren't Persons': A Survey of Delayed Personhood. In H. Otto & H. Keller (Eds). *Different Faces of Attachment: Cultural Variations of a Universal Human Need* (66–112). Cambridge University Press.

12. H. Otto (2014). Don't Show Your Emotions! Emotion Regulation and Attachment in the Cameroonian Nso. In H. Otto & H. Keller (Eds). *Different Faces of Attachment: Cultural Variations on a Universal Human Need* (215–29). Cambridge University Press.

13. D. F. Lancy (2022). *The Anthropology of Childhood: Cherubs, Chattel, Changelings* (3rd ed.). Cambridge University Press.

14. K. Hastrup (1992). A Question of Reason: Breast-Feeding Patterns in Seventeenth- and Eighteenth-Century Iceland. In V. Maher (Ed.). *The Anthropology of Breast-Feeding: Natural Law or Social Construct?* (91–108). Berg.

15. J. L. Martucci (2015). *Back to the Breast: Natural Motherhood and Breastfeeding in America*. University of Chicago Press.

16. D. Wiessinger, D. West & T. Pitman (2010). The *Womanly Art of Breastfeeding* (8th ed.). Ballantine Books.

17. J. D. Ward (2000). *La Leche League: At the Crossroads of Medicine, Feminism and Religion*. University of North Carolina Press.

18. A. Freeman (2017). Unmothering Black Women: Formula Feeding as an Incident of Slavery. *Hastings LJ, 69*, 1545.

19. Nash, 2021.

20. S. DeVane-Johnson, C. W. Giscombe, R. Williams II, et al. (2018). A Qualitative Study of Social, Cultural, and Historical Influences on African American Women's Infant-Feeding Practices. *The Journal of Perinatal Education*, 27(2), 71–85.

21. L. M. Blum (1999). *At the Breast: Ideologies of Breastfeeding and Motherhood in the Contemporary United States.* Beacon Press.

22. P. Salzman-Mitchell (2012). Tenderness or Taboo: Images of Breast-Feeding Mothers in Greek and Latin Literature. In P. Salzman-Mitchell & L. H. Petersen (Eds). *Mothering and Motherhood in Ancient Greece and Rome* (141–64). University of Texas Press.

23. E. Badinter (1981). *The Myth of Motherhood: An Historical View of the Maternal Instinct.* Souvenir Press (E & A).

24. E. J. Unsworth (2021). *After the Storm: Postnatal Depression and the Utter Weirdness of New Motherhood.* Profile Books.

25. See for example Centers for Disease Control and Prevention (2024). *Rates of Any and Exclusive Breastfeeding by Socio-demographics Among Children Born in 2020.* F. McAndrew, J. Thompson, L. Fellows, et al. (2012). *Infant Feeding Survey 2010.* Health and Social Care Information Centre.

26. O. Avishai (2011). Managing the Lactating Body: The Breastfeeding Project in the Age of Anxiety. In P. Liamputtong (Ed.). *Infant Feeding Practices: A Cross-Cultural Perspective* (23–38). Springer.

27. C. T. Beck & S. Watson (2008). Impact of Birth Trauma on Breast-Feeding: A Tale of Two Pathways. *Nursing Research, 57*(4), 228–36.

28. L. A. Tarasoff (2018). *A Qualitative Study of Embodiment Among Women with Physical Disabilities During the Perinatal Period and Early Motherhood.* Doctoral Dissertation, University of Toronto.

29. D. Williams, J. Webber, B. Pell, et al. (2019). 'Nobody Knows, or Seems to Know How Rheumatology and Breastfeeding Works': Women's Experiences of Breastfeeding Whilst Managing a Long-Term Limiting Condition – A Qualitative Visual Methods Study. *Midwifery, 78*, 91–6.

30. Unsworth, 2021.

31. S. Símonardóttir (2016). Getting the Green Light: Experiences of Icelandic Mothers Struggling with Breastfeeding. *Sociological Research Online, 21*(4), 1–13.

32. S. Knaak (2005). Breast-Feeding, Bottle-Feeding and Dr. Spock: The Shifting Context of Choice. *Canadian Review of Sociology/Revue Canadienne de Sociologie, 42*(2), 197–216.

33. A. Brown (2016). *Breastfeeding Uncovered: Who Really Decides How We Feed Our Babies?* Pinter & Martin.
34. ComRes (2019). BBC Radio Sheffield & BBC *Woman's Hour* – Feeding Your Baby Poll, January 2019. *Online.*
35. E. Odom, R. Li, K. S. Scanlon, et al. (2013). Reasons for Earlier than Desired Cessation of Breastfeeding. *Pediatrics, 131*(3), 726–32.
36. McAndrew, Thompson, Fellows, et al., 2012.
37. Mumsnet (2017). Barriers to Breastfeeding: The Reasons Why Women Stop Breastfeeding. *Online.*
38. S. Komninou, V. Fallon, J. C. G. Halford & J. A. Harrold (2017). Differences in the Emotional and Practical Experiences of Exclusively Breastfeeding and Combination Feeding Mothers. *Maternal & Child Nutrition, 13*(3).
39. Birthrights (2022). *Systemic Racism, Not Broken Bodies: An Inquiry into Racial Injustice and Human Rights in UK Maternity Care.*
40. V. Bhavnani & M. Newburn (2010). *Left to Your Own Devices: The Postnatal Care Experiences of 1260 First-Time Mothers.* NCT.
41. Thomson, Ebisch-Burton & Flacking, 2014.
42. See for example UNICEF UK (2024). Overcoming Breastfeeding Problems: Low Milk Supply. *Online.*
43. NHS (2024). Breastfeeding: The First Few Days. *Online.*
44. Australian Institute of Health and Welfare (2011). *2010 Australian National Infant Feeding Survey.* McAndrew, Thompson, Fellows, et al., 2012.
45. Odom, Li, Scanlon, et al., 2013.
46. R. M. Powell, M. Mitra, S. C. Smeltzer, et al. (2018). Breastfeeding Among Women with Physical Disabilities in the United States. *Journal of Human Lactation, 34*(2), 253–61.
47. P. Pearson-Glaze (2021, 22 June). Reasons for Low Milk Supply. *Breastfeeding Support.* D. Cassar-Uhl (2023, 22 November). *Hypoplasia/Insufficient Glandular Tissue.* KellyMom.
48. M. R. Neifert (2001). Prevention of Breastfeeding Tragedies. *Pediatric Clinics of North America, 48,* 273–97.
49. A. M. Stuebe, B. J. Horton, E. Chetwynd, et al. (2014). Prevalence and Risk Factors for Early, Undesired Weaning Attributed to Lactation Dysfunction. *Journal of Women's Health, 23*(5), 404–12.
50. Brown, 2016.
51. Stuebe, Horton, Chetwynd, et al., 2014.
52. NHS (2024). Breastfeeding: Is My Baby Getting Enough Milk? *Online.*
53. National Institute for Health and Care Excellence (2022). Scenario: Breastfeeding Problems – Management. *Online.*

54. E. Kasket (2019, 11 February). 'Breast Is Best' Nearly Cost My Baby Her Life. *Medium*.

55. C. del Castillo-Hegyi (2015, 18 April). Letter to Doctors and Parents About the Dangers of Insufficient Exclusive Breastfeeding. *The Fed Is Best Foundation*.

56. C. Criado Perez (2019). *Invisible Women: Exposing Data Bias in a World Designed for Men*. Chatto & Windus.

57. A. N. Bazzano, R. Hofer, S. Thibeau, et al. (2016). A Review of Herbal and Pharmaceutical Galactagogues for Breast-Feeding. *Ochsner Journal*, *16*(4), 511–24.

58. C. M. Ndikom, B. Fawole & R. E. Ilesanmi (2014). Extra Fluids for Breastfeeding Mothers for Increasing Milk Production. *Cochrane Database of Systematic Reviews*, (6).

59. I. Zakarija-Grkovic & F. Stewart (2020). Treatments for Breast Engorgement During Lactation. *Cochrane Database of Systematic Reviews*, (9).

60. A. Brown (2019, 11 March). Quit Telling Women Breastfeeding Is an Optional Lifestyle Choice. *The Conversation*.

61. J. B. Wolf (2011). *Is Breast Best? Taking on the Breastfeeding Experts and the New High Stakes of Motherhood*. New York University Press.

62. E. Oster (2019). *Cribsheet: A Data-Driven Guide to Better, More Relaxed Parenting, from Birth to Preschool*. Penguin Press.

63. C. G. Victora, R. Bahl, A. J. Barros, et al. (2016). Breastfeeding in the 21st Century: Epidemiology, Mechanisms, and Lifelong Effect. *The Lancet*, *387*, 475–90.

64. World Health Organization (2024). Breastfeeding. *Online*.

65. See for example G. Der, G. D. Batty & I. J. Deary (2006). Effect of Breast Feeding on Intelligence in Children: Prospective Study, Sibling Pairs Analysis, and Meta-Analysis. *BMJ*, *333*.

66. C. G. Colen & D. M. Ramey (2014). Is Breast Truly Best? Estimating the Effects of Breastfeeding on Long-Term Child Health and Wellbeing in the United States Using Sibling Comparisons. *Social Science & Medicine*, *109*, 55–65. A. Brown (2019). *Informed is Best: How to Spot Fake News About Your Pregnancy, Birth and Baby*. Pinter & Martin.

67. Victora, Bahl, Barros, et al., 2016.

68. The All-Party Parliamentary Group on Infant Feeding and Inequalities (2018). *Inquiry into the Cost of Infant Formula in the United Kingdom*.

69. Palmer, 2009.

70. K. Sikkink (1986). Codes of Conduct for Transnational Corporations: The Case of the WHO/UNICEF Code. *International Organization*, *40*(4), 815–40.

71. S. Kitzinger (1987). *The Experience of Breastfeeding* (2nd ed.). Penguin.

72. See for example Save the Children (2018). *Don't Push It: Why the Formula Milk Industry Must Clean Up its Act.* World Health Organization (2022). *How the Marketing of Formula Milk Influences Our Decisions on Infant Feeding.*

73. UNICEF UK (2014). Guidelines on Providing Information for Parents About Formula Feeding. *UNICEF UK Infosheet.*

74. Thomson, Ebisch-Burton & Flacking, 2014.

75. B. M Lagan, A. Symon, J. Dalzell & H. Whitford (2014). 'The Midwives Aren't Allowed to Tell You': Perceived Infant Feeding Policy Restrictions in a Formula Feeding Culture–The Feeding Your Baby Study. *Midwifery*, 30(3), 49–55.

76. NHS (2024). How to Stop Breastfeeding. *Online.*

77. See for example Association of Breastfeeding Mothers (2024). Questions Mums Ask About Stopping Breastfeeding. *Online.*

78. La Leche League GB (2016). Thinking of Weaning? *Online.*

79. R. L. Trivers (1974). Parent-Offspring Conflict. *Integrative and Comparative Biology*, 14(1), 249–64.

80. L. Minturn & W. W. Lambert (1964). *Mothers of Six Cultures: Antecedents of Child Rearing.* John Wiley.

81. E. Homewood, A. Tweed, M. Cree & J. Crossley (2009). Becoming Occluded: The Transition to Motherhood of Women with Postnatal Depression. *Qualitative Research in Psychology*, 6(4), 313–29.

82. Thomson, Ebisch-Burton & Flacking, 2014.

83. V. Fallon, S. Komninou, K. M. Bennett, et al. (2017). The Emotional and Practical Experiences of Formula-Feeding Mothers. *Maternal & Child Nutrition*, 13(4).

84. A. Grant (2016). 'I . . . Don't Want to See You Flashing Your Bits Around': Exhibitionism, Othering and Good Motherhood. *Geoforum*, 71, 52–61.

85. S. Kitzinger (2005) *The Politics of Birth.* Elsevier.

86. YouGov (2013). No Breastfeeding in the Swimming Pool. *Online.*

87. A. Sheehan, K. Gribble & V. Schmied (2019). It's Okay to Breastfeed in Public But . . . *International Breastfeeding Journal*, 14(24), 1–11.

88. Thomson, Ebisch-Burton & Flacking, 2014.

89. K. L. Newman & I. R. Williamson (2018). 'Why Aren't You Stopping Now?!' Exploring Accounts of White Women Breastfeeding Beyond Six Months in the East of England, *Appetite*, 129, 228–35.

90. C. Faircloth (2013). *Militant Lactivism? Attachment Parenting and Intensive Motherhood in the UK and France.* Berghahn Books.

91. P. Hamilton (2021). *Black Mothers and Attachment Parenting: A Black Feminist Analysis of Intensive Mothering in Britain and Canada.* Bristol University Press.

92. Freeman, 2017.
93. NCT (2018). *Infant Feeding Message Framework: Values and Approaches to Infant Feeding Support.*
94. J. P. Grant (1985). *The State of the World's Children 1985.* Oxford University Press.
95. See for example National Maternity Review (2016). *Better Births: Improving Outcomes of Maternity Services in England.*
96. Public Health England & UNICEF UK (2016). *Commissioning Infant Feeding Services: A Toolkit for Local Authorities (Part 2).*
97. K. Kendall-Tackett (2015). The New Paradigm for Depression in New Mothers: Current Findings on Maternal Depression, Breastfeeding and Resiliency Across the Lifespan. *Breastfeeding Review, 23(1),* 7–10.
98. V. Maher (1992). Breast-Feeding and Maternal Depletion: Natural Law or Cultural Arrangements. In V. Maher (Ed.). *The Anthropology of Breast-Feeding: Natural Law or Social Construct?* (151–80). Berg.
99. UNICEF UK (2016). Call to Action on Infant Feeding in the UK. *Online.*
100. Royal College of Midwives (2019, 27 January). RCM Responds to BBC Poll on Women's Experiences of Breastfeeding. *Online.*
101. Kitzinger, 1987.
102. K. Williams, N. Donaghue & T. Kurz (2012). 'Giving Guilt the Flick'? An Investigation of Mothers' Talk About Guilt in Relation to Infant Feeding. *Psychology of Women Quarterly, 37(1),* 97–112.
103. F. Woollard (2019). Requirements to Justify Breastfeeding in Public: A Philosophical Analysis. *International Breastfeeding Journal, 14,* 26.
104. The Royal College of Midwives (2018). *Position Statement: Infant Feeding.*
105. T. MacDonald, J. Noel-Weiss, D. West, et al. (2016). Transmasculine Individuals' Experiences with Lactation, Chestfeeding, and Gender Identity: A Qualitative Study. *BMC Pregnancy and Childbirth, 16,* 106.
106. A. McFadden, A. Gavine, M. J. Renfrew, et al. (2017). Support for Healthy Breastfeeding Mothers with Healthy Term Babies. *Cochrane Database of Systematic Reviews, (2).*
107. Brown, 2016.
108. R. L. Spencer, S. Greatrex-White & D. M. Fraser (2015). 'I Thought It Would Keep Them All Quiet.' Women's Experiences of Breastfeeding as Illusions of Compliance: An Interpretive Phenomenological Study. *Journal of Advanced Nursing, 71(5),* 1076–86.

5. Attachment Issues

1. R. Duschinsky (2020). *Cornerstones of Attachment Research*. Oxford University Press.
2. J. Bowlby (1958). *Can I Leave My Baby?* National Association for Mental Health.
3. S. Van Dijken (1998). *John Bowlby, His Early Life: A Biographical Journey into the Roots of Attachment Theory*. Free Association Books.
4. R. Karen (1994). *Becoming Attached: First Relationships and How They Shape Our Capacity to Love*. Oxford University Press.
5. S. Freud (1938). *An Outline of Psychoanalysis*. Hogarth Press. J. Bowlby (1958). The Nature of the Child's Tie to His Mother. *The International Journal of Psycho-Analysis, 39*, 350–73. M. D. S. Ainsworth (1969). Object Relations, Dependency, and Attachment: A Theoretical Review of the Infant-Mother Relationship. *Child Development, 40*, 969–1025.
6. J. Bowlby (1953). *Child Care and the Growth of Love*. Penguin.
7. H. McCarthy (2020). *Double Lives: A History of Working Motherhood*. Bloomsbury.
8. A. Cuthbert (1948). *Housewife Baby Book*. Hulton Press.
9. A. Cuthbert (1955). *Housewife Baby Book* (2nd ed.). Hulton Press.
10. Cited in M. Vicedo (2013). *The Nature and Nurture of Love: From Imprinting to Attachment in Cold War America*. University of Chicago Press.
11. M. D. Ainsworth, R. G. Andry, R. G. Harlow, et al. (1962). *Deprivation of Maternal Care: A Reassessment of its Effects*. World Health Organization.
12. B. Wootton (1962). A Social Scientist's Approach to Maternal Deprivation. In *Deprivation of Maternal Care: A Reassessment of its Effects* (63–73). World Health Organization.
13. J. Bowlby (1969). *Attachment and Loss: Attachment (Volume 1)*. The Hogarth Press and the Institute of Pscyho-analysis.
14. V. Hunter (1991). John Bowlby: An Interview by Virginia Hunter. *Psychoanalytic Review, 78*(2), 159–75.
15. S. B. Hrdy (2011). *Mothers and Others: The Evolutionary Origins of Mutual Understanding*. Harvard University Press.
16. J. Bowlby (1988). *A Secure Base: Parent-Child Attachment and Healthy Human Development*. Basic Books.
17. Bowlby, 1969.
18. S. Freud (2004). *Civilisation and its Discontents*. Penguin Books.
19. Interview with Robert Karen quoted in Karen, 1994.
20. Duschinsky, 2020.
21. M. D. S. Ainsworth (1983). Mary D. Salter Ainsworth. In A. N. O'Connell & N. F. Russo (Eds). *Models Of Achievement: Reflections of Eminent Women in Psychology* (200–19). Columbia University Press.

22. McCarthy, 2020.

23. R. A. LeVine (2014). Attachment Theory as Cultural Ideology. In H. Otto & H. Keller (Eds). *Different Faces of Attachment: Cultural Variations on a Universal Human Need*, (50–65). Cambridge University Press.

24. M. Shapira (2013). *The War Inside: Psychoanalysis, Total War, and the Making of the Democratic Self in Postwar Britain*. Cambridge University Press.

25. Karen, 1994.

26. Bowlby, 1953.

27. Community Affairs References Committee (2012). *Commonwealth Contribution to Former Forced Adoption Policies and Practices*. Parliament House.

28. S. Moullin, J. Waldfogel & E. Washbrook (2014). *Baby Bonds: Parenting, Attachment and a Secure Base for Children*. Sutton Trust.

29. Vicedo, 2013.

30. Bowlby, 1969.

31. J. Robertson & J. Robertson (1971). Young Children in Brief Separation: A Fresh Look. *The Psychoanalytic Study of the Child*, 26(1), 264–315.

32. Vicedo, 2013.

33. Ainsworth, 1983.

34. J. Bowlby, M. Ainsworth, M. Boston & D. Rosenbluth (1956). The Effects of Mother-Child Separation: A Follow-up Study. *The British Journal of Medical Psychology*, 29, 211–47.

35. L. van Rosmalen, F. C. van der Horst & R. van der Veer (2016). From Secure Dependency to Attachment: Mary Ainsworth's Integration of Blatz's Security Theory into Bowlby's Attachment Theory. *History of Psychology*, 19(1), 22–39.

36. M. D. S. Ainsworth, S. M. Bell & D. J. Stayton (1971). Individual Differences in Strange-Situation Behavior of One-Year-Olds. In H. R. Schaffer (Ed.). *The Origins of Human Social Relations* (17–58). Academic Press.

37. Karen, 1994.

38. Ainsworth, 1983.

39. Vicedo, 2013.

40. Ainsworth, Bell & Stayton, 1971.

41. M. D. S. Ainsworth & B. A. Wittig (1969). Attachment and the Exploratory Behaviour of One-Year-Olds in a Strange Situation. In B. M. Foss (Ed.). *Determinants of Infant Behaviour*, 4 (113–36). Methuen.

42. M. D. S. Ainsworth, M. C. Blehar, E. Waters & S. N. Wall (1978). *Patterns of Attachment: A Psychological Study of the Strange Situation*. Psychology Press.

43. Ainsworth, Bell & Stayton, 1971.
44. Ibid.
45. Karen, 1994.
46. M. E. Lamb, R. A. Thompson, W. P. Gardner, et al. (1984). Security of Infantile Attachment as Assessed in the 'Strange Situation': Its Study and Biological Interpretation. *Behavioral and Brain Sciences*, 7(1), 127–47.
47. Karen, 1994.
48. I. Bretherton (2003). Mary Ainsworth: Insightful Observer and Courageous Theoretician. G. A. Kimble & M. Wertheimer (Eds). In *Portraits of Pioneers in Psychology*, 5 (317–31). Psychology Press.
49. E. P. Davis & L. M. Glynn (2024). Annual Research Review: The Power of Predictability – Patterns of Signals in Early Life Shape Neurodevelopment and Mental Health Trajectories. *Journal of Child Psychology and Psychiatry*, 65(4), 508–34.
50. D. Wastell & S. White (2017). *Blinded by Science: The Social Implications of Epigenetics and Neuroscience.* Policy Press.
51. World Health Organization (2018). *Nurturing Care for Early Childhood Development: A Framework for Helping Children Survive and Thrive to Transform Health and Human Potential.*
52. The First 1001 Days (2021). *An Age of Opportunity (Evidence Brief 1).*
53. M. D. S. Ainsworth, S. M. Bell & D. J. Stayton (1974) Infant-Mother Attachment and Social Development: 'Socialisation' as Products of Reciprocal Responsiveness to Signals. In M. P. M. Richards (Ed.). *The Integration of a Child into a Social World* (99–135). Cambridge University Press.
54. Bowlby, 1988.
55. Bowlby, 1958.
56. Moullin, Waldfogel & Washbrook, 2014.
57. The Social Mobility Commission (2017). *Helping Parents to Parent.*
58. Ainsworth, Bell, Stayton, 1971.
59. M. S. De Wolff & M. H. Van IJzendoorn (1997). Sensitivity and Attachment: A Meta-Analysis on Parental Antecedents of Infant Attachment. *Child Development*, 68(4), 571–91.
60. N. Lucassen, A. Tharner, M. H. Van IJzendoorn, et al. (2011). The Association Between Paternal Sensitivity and Infant–Father Attachment Security: A Meta-Analysis of Three Decades of Research. *Journal of Family Psychology*, 25(6), 986–92.
61. NICHD Early Child Care Research Network (1997). The Effects of Infant Child Care on Infant-Mother Attachment Security: Results of the NICHD Study of Early Child Care. *Child Development*, 68(5), 860–79.

62. M. Main & J. Solomon (1986). Discovery of a New, Insecure-Disorganized/Disoriented Attachment Pattern. In M. Yogman & T. B. Brazelton (Eds). *Affective Development in Infancy* (195–24). Ablex. C. Cyr, E. M. Euser, M. J. Bakermans-Kranenburg & M. H. Van IJzendoorn (2010). Attachment Security and Disorganization in Maltreating and High-Risk Families: A Series of Meta-Analyses. *Development and Psychopathology*, 22(1), 87–108.

63. E. Longhi, L. Murray, D. Wellsted, et al. (2019). *Minding the Baby® Home-Visiting Programme for Vulnerable Young Mothers: Results of a Randomised Controlled Trial in the UK*. NSPCC.

64. J. Mesman & R. A. Emmen (2013). Mary Ainsworth's Legacy: A Systematic Review of Observational Instruments Measuring Parental Sensitivity. *Attachment & Human Development*, 15(5–6), 485–506.

65. R. A. LeVine (2014). Attachment Theory as Cultural Ideology. In H. Otto & H. Keller (Eds). *Different Faces of Attachment: Cultural Variations on a Universal Human Need*, (50–65). Cambridge University Press.

66. D. R. Pederson, G. Moran & S. Bento (1999). Maternal Behaviour Q-sort Version 3.1. *Psychology Publications*, Paper 1.

67. LeVine, 2014

68. Duschinsky, 2020.

69. S. S. Woodhouse (2019, 28 May). Being a 'Good Enough' Parent is Actually a Great Thing, New Research Shows. *Thrive Global*.

70. S. S. Woodhouse, J. R. Scott, A. D. Hepworth & J. Cassidy (2020). Secure Base Provision: A New Approach to Examining Links Between Maternal Caregiving and Infant Attachment. *Child Development*, 91(1), 249–65.

71. G. Scheidecker, N. Chaudhary, H. Keller, et al. (2023). 'Poor Brain Development' in the Global South? Challenging the Science of Early Childhood Interventions. *Ethos*, 51(1), 3–26.

72. C. Cuthbert, G. Rayns & K. Stanley (2011). *All Babies Count: Prevention and Protection for Vulnerable Babies*. NSPCC.

73. Bowlby, 1988.

74. R. A. Thompson (2016). Early Attachment and Later Development: Reframing the Questions. In J. Cassidy & P. R. Shaver (Eds). *Handbook of Attachment: Theory, Research, and Clinical Applications* (330–48) (3rd ed.). Guilford Press.

75. C. Howes & S. Spieker (2016). Attachment Relationships in the Context of Multiple Caregivers. In J. Cassidy & P. R. Shaver (Eds). *Handbook of Attachment: Theory, Research, and Clinical Applications* (314–29) (3rd ed.). Guilford Press.

76. L. A. Sroufe (2016). The Place of Attachment in Development. In J. Cassidy & P. R. Shaver (Eds). *Handbook of Attachment: Theory, Research, and Clinical Applications* (997–1011) (3rd ed.). Guilford Press.
77. S. Pinker (2009). Foreword. In J. R. Harris. *The Nurture Assumption: Why Children Turn Out the Way They Do* (2nd ed.). Simon & Schuster.
78. Moullin, Waldfogel & Washbrook, 2014.
79. Duschinsky, 2020.
80. E. Meins (2016, 25 November). Overrated: The Predictive Power of Attachment. *The Psychologist.*
81. Moullin, Waldfogel & Washbrook, 2014.
82. V. Gillies, R. Edwards & N. Horsley (2017). *Challenging the Politics of Early Intervention: Who's 'Saving' Children and Why.* Policy Press.
83. Wave Trust (2013). *Conception to Age 2 – The Age of Opportunity.*
84. See for example Bowlby, 1969.
85. T. Forslund, P. Granqvist, M. H. Van IJzendoorn, et al. (2022). Attachment Goes to Court: Child Protection and Custody Issues. *Attachment & Human Development,* 24(1), 1–52.
86. P. Granqvist, L. A. Sroufe, M. Dozier, et al. (2017). Disorganized Attachment in Infancy: A Review of the Phenomenon and its Implications for Clinicians and Policy-Makers. *Attachment & Human Development,* 19(6), 534–58.
87. Bowlby, 1988.
88. M. Pinquart, C. Feußner & L. Ahnert (2013). Meta-Analytic Evidence for Stability in Attachments from Infancy to Early Adulthood. *Attachment & Human Development,* 15(2), 189–218.
89. L. A. Sroufe, B. Coffino & E. A. Carlson (2010). Conceptualizing the Role of Early Experience: Lessons from the Minnesota Longitudinal Study. *Developmental Review,* 30(1), 36–51.
90. Sroufe, 2016.
91. Bowlby, 1969.
92. Vicedo, 2013.
93. G. Kochanska & S. Kim (2013). Early Attachment Organization with Both Parents and Future Behavior Problems: From Infancy to Middle Childhood. *Child Development,* 84(1), 283–96.
94. Wave Trust, 2013.
95. S. B. Hrdy (2001, May). Mothers and Others. *Natural History.*
96. J. Mesman, T. Minter & A. Angnged (2016). Received Sensitivity: Adapting Ainsworth's Scale to Capture Sensitivity in a Multiple-Caregiver Context. *Attachment & Human Development,* 18(2), 101–14.
97. B. Röttger-Rössler (2014). Bonding and Belonging Beyond WEIRD Worlds: Rethinking Attachment Theory on the Basis of Cross-Cultural

Anthropological Data. In H. Otto & H. Keller (Eds). *Different Faces of Attachment: Cultural Variations on a Universal Human Need* (141–68). Cambridge University Press.

98. Hrdy, 2011.
99. A. Gopnik (2016). *The Gardener and the Carpenter: What the New Science of Child Development Tells Us About the Relationship Between Parents and Children*. The Bodley Head.
100. Bowlby, 1953.
101. K. Pickert (2012, 10 May). Meet Dr. Bill Sears, the Man Who Remade Motherhood. *Time*.
102. W. Sears & M. Sears (2001). *The Attachment Parenting Book: A Commonsense Guide to Understanding and Nurturing Your Baby*. Little, Brown.
103. P. Hamilton (2021). *Black Mothers and Attachment Parenting: A Black Feminist Analysis of Intensive Mothering in Britain and Canada*. Bristol University Press.
104. World Economic Forum (2023). *Global Gender Gap Report: 2023*.
105. S. Símonardóttir (2016). Constructing the Attached Mother in the 'World's Most Feminist Country'. *Women's Studies International Forum*, 56, 103–12.
106. Gillies, Edwards & Horsley, 2017.
107. Office for Health Improvement and Disparities (2022). Healthy Beginnings: Applying All Our Health. *Online*.
108. The Scottish Government (2012). *National Parenting Strategy: Making a Positive Difference to Children and Young People Through Parenting*.
109. Welsh Government (2022). *An Overview of the Healthy Child Wales Programme*.
110. M. De Klyen & M. T. Greenberg (2016). Attachment and Psychopathology in Childhood. In J. Cassidy & P. R. Shaver (Eds). *Handbook of Attachment: Theory, Research, and Clinical Applications* (639–66) (3rd ed.). Guilford Press.
111. B. Wright, M. Barry, E. Hughes, et al. (2015). Clinical Effectiveness and Cost-Effectiveness of Parenting Interventions for Children with Severe Attachment Problems: A Systematic Review and Meta-Analysis. *Health Technology Assessment*, 19(52), vii–xxviii.
112. Bowlby, 1988.
113. S. M. Bell & M. D. S. Ainsworth (1972). Infant Crying and Maternal Responsiveness. *Child Development*, 43(4), 1171–90.
114. H. Keller (2014). Introduction: Understanding Relationships – What We Would Need to Know to Conceptualize Attachment as the Cultural Solution of a Universal Developmental Task. In H. Otto & H. Keller

(Eds). *Different Faces of Attachment: Cultural Variations on a Universal Human Need* (1–24). Cambridge University Press.

115. V. J. Carlson & R. L. Harwood (2014). The Precursors of Attachment Security: Behavioral Systems and Culture. In H. Otto & H. Keller (Eds). *Different Faces of Attachment: Cultural Variations on a Universal Human Need* (278–303). Cambridge University Press.

116. S. White, M. Gibson, D. Wastell & P. Walsh (2020). *Reassessing Attachment Theory in Child Welfare: A Critical Appraisal.* Policy Press.

6. Babies Don't Need to Be Built

1. S. Harkness, C. M. Super, R. Moises, et al. (2010). Parental Ethnotheories of Children's Learning. In D. F. Lancy, J. Bock & S. Gaskins (Eds) (2010). *The Anthropology of Learning in Childhood* (65–81). Rowman & Littlefield.

2. S. Atzil, T. Hendler & R. Feldman (2011). Specifying the Neurobiological Basis of Human Attachment: Brain, Hormones, and Behavior in Synchronous and Intrusive Mothers. *Neuropsychopharmacology,* 36(13), 2603–15.

3. H. Keller (2014). Introduction: Understanding Relationships – What We Would Need to Know to Conceptualize Attachment as the Cultural Solution of a Universal Developmental Task. In H. Otto & H. Keller (Eds). *Different Faces of Attachment: Cultural Variations on a Universal Human Need* (1–24). Cambridge University Press.

4. A. Turmel (2008). *A Historical Sociology of Childhood: Developmental Thinking, Categorisation and Graphic Visualisation.* Cambridge University Press.

5. A. Easter & M. Newburn (2015). *From Babies to Toddlers: First-Time Mothers' and Fathers' Experiences from a Longitudinal Study. First 1,001 Days Final Study Report.* NCT.

6. M. Sunderland (2016). *What Every Parent Needs to Know: Love, Nurture and Play with Your Child* (2nd ed.). Dorling Kindersley.

7. P. K. Smith, H. Cowie & M. Blades (2015). *Understanding Children's Development* (6th ed.). Wiley.

8. A. Gopnik (2016). *The Gardener and the Carpenter: What the New Science of Child Development Tells Us About the Relationship Between Parents and Children.* The Bodley Head.

9. D. F. Lancy (2022). *The Anthropology of Childhood: Cherubs, Chattel, Changelings* (3rd ed.). Cambridge University Press.

10. G. Cross (2015). Play, Games, and Toys. In P. S. Fass (Ed.). *The Routledge History of Childhood in the Western World* (267–82). Routledge.

11. J. Golden & L. Weiner (2011). Reading Baby Books: Medicine, Marketing, Money and the Lives of American Infants. *Journal of Social History*, 44(3), 667–87.

12. R. D. Apple (1987). *Mothers and Medicine: A Social History of Infant Feeding, 1890–1950*. University of Wisconsin Press.

13. L. E. Holt (1907). *The Care and Feeding of Children: A Catechism for the Use of Mothers and Children's Nurses* (4th ed.). D. Appleton.

14. M. Wolfenstein (1998). Fun Morality: An Analysis of Recent Child-Training Literature. In H. Jenkins (Ed.). *Childhood in Contemporary Cultures* (199–208). New York University Press.

15. P. N. Stearns (2003). *Anxious Parents: A History of Modern Childrearing in America*. New York University Press.

16. R. Parker (2005). *Torn in Two: The Experience of Maternal Ambivalence* (2nd ed.). Virago.

17. Sunderland, 2016.

18. A. Combe & J. Clark (1860). *The Management of Infancy: Physiological and Moral*. Kessinger Legacy Reprints.

19. S. Frankenburg (1946). *Common Sense in the Nursery* (3rd ed.). Penguin.

20. S. Lassonde (2015). Age, Schooling, and Development. In P. S. Fass (Ed.). *The Routledge History of Childhood in the Western World* (211–28). Routledge.

21. V. A. Zelizer (1985). *Pricing the Priceless Child: The Changing Social Value of Children*. Basic Books.

22. J. Grant (2015). Parent–Child Relations in Western Europe and North America, 1500–Present. In P. S. Fass (Ed.). *The Routledge History of Childhood in the Western World* (103–24). Routledge.

23. B. Spock (1946). *The Common Sense Book of Baby and Child Care*. Duell, Sloan and Pearce. B. Spock & S. J. Parker (1998). *Dr. Spock's Baby and Child Care* (7th ed.). Pocket Books.

24. B. Spock (1957). *Baby & Child Care*. The Bodley Head. Spock & Parker (1998).

25. T. Maier (1998). *Dr Spock: An American Life*. Harcourt Brace.

26. UNICEF UK (2023). *Building a Happy Baby: A Guide for Parents*.

27. J. Chan (2022). *The School for Good Mothers*. Penguin Books.

28. National Scientific Council on the Developing Child (2007). *The Timing and Quality of Early Experiences Combine to Shape Brain Architecture*. Center on the Developing Child, Harvard University.

29. National Scientific Council on the Developing Child (2007). *The Science of Early Childhood Development: Closing the Gap Between What We Know and What We Do*. Center on the Developing Child, Harvard University.

30. Center on the Developing Child (2024). Serve & Return Interaction Shapes Brain Circuitry. *Online*.
31. H. Rose & S. Rose (2016). *Can Neuroscience Change Our Minds?* John Wiley & Sons.
32. M. Cobb (2020). *The Idea of the Brain: A History*. Profile Books.
33. K. J. Mitchell (2018). *Innate: How the Wiring of Our Brains Shapes Who We Are*. Princeton University Press.
34. Vroom (2024). Sharing the Science of Early Brain Development.
35. NSPCC (2019). *Look, Say, Sing, Play to Build Your Baby's Brain Every Day*.
36. NSPCC (2024). Just Remember to Look, Say, Sing, Play.
37. Sunderland, 2016.
38. E. R. Moore, G. C. Anderson, N. Bergman & T. Dowswell (2012). Early Skin-To-Skin Contact for Mothers and Their Healthy Newborn Infants. *Cochrane Database of Systematic Reviews*, *5*(3).
39. K. L. Raby, G. I. Roisman, R. C. Fraley & J. A. Simpson (2015). The Enduring Predictive Significance of Early Maternal Sensitivity: Social and Academic Competence through Age 32 years. *Child Development*, *86*(3), 695–708.
40. M. A. Hofer (1996). On the Nature and Consequences of Early Loss. *Psychosomatic Medicine*, *58*(6), 570–81. K. M. Kramer, B. S. Cushing & C. S. Carter (2003). Developmental Effects of Oxytocin on Stress Response: Single Versus Repeated Exposure. *Physiology & Behavior*, *79*(4–5), 775–82. P. Buckley, R. S. Rigda, L. Mundy & I. McMillen (2002). Interaction Between Bed Sharing and Other Sleep Environments During the First Six Months of Life. *Early Human Development*, *66*(2), 123–32.
41. A. H. Veenema (2009). Early Life Stress, the Development of Aggression and Neuroendocrine and Neurobiological Correlates: What Can We Learn from Animal Models? *Frontiers in Neuroendocrinology*, *30*(4), 497–518.
42. Quoted in S. Poole (2012, 6 September). Your Brain on Pseudoscience: The Rise of Popular Neurobollocks. *New Statesman*.
43. D. Wastell & S. White (2017). *Blinded by Science: The Social Implications of Epigenetics and Neuroscience*. Policy Press.
44. T. Jensen (2018). *Parenting the Crisis: The Cultural Politics of Parent-Blame*. Policy Press.
45. See for example K. M. Robson & R. Kumar (1980). Delayed Onset of Maternal Affection after Childbirth. *The British Journal of Psychiatry*, *136*(4), 347–53.
46. H. Ball & P. S. Blair (2021). *The Health Professional's Guide to: 'Caring for Your Baby at Night'*. UNICEF UK.

47. J. Macvarish (2023). Babies' Brains and Parenting Policy: The Insensitive Mother. In E. Lee, J. Bristow, C. Faircloth & J. Macvarish. *Parenting Culture Studies* (215–39) (2nd ed.). Palgrave Macmillan.

48. V. Gillies, R. Edwards & N. Horsley (2017). *Challenging the Politics of Early Intervention: Who's 'Saving' Children and Why*. Policy Press.

49. First 1001 Days All-Party Parliamentary Group (2015). *Building Great Britons: Conception to Age 2*.

50. Gillies, Edwards & Horsley, 2017.

51. R. Brown & H. Ward (2013). *Decision-Making within a Child's Timeframe: An Overview of Current Research Evidence for Family Justice Professionals Concerning Child Development and the Impact of Maltreatment*. Childhood Wellbeing Research Centre.

52. Wastell & White, 2017.

53. World Health Organization (2018). *Nurturing Care for Early Childhood Development: A Framework for Helping Children Survive and Thrive to Transform Health and Human Potential*.

54. G. Scheidecker, N. Chaudhary, H. Keller, et al. (2023). 'Poor Brain Development' in the Global South? Challenging the Science of Early Childhood Interventions. *Ethos*, *51*(1), 3–26.

55. Gillies, Edwards & Horsley, 2017.

56. Saving Brains (2024). Family-Inclusive Early Brain Stimulation (FInE BrainS). *Online*.

57. National Scientific Council on the Developing Child (2007). *The Science of Early Childhood Development: Closing the Gap Between What We Know and What We Do*. Center on the Developing Child, Harvard University. M. J. Meaney (2001). Maternal Care, Gene Expression, and the Transmission of Individual Differences in Stress Reactivity Across Generations. *Annual Review of Neuroscience*, *24*(1), 1161–92.

58. A. Gopnik, A. N. Meltzoff and P. K. Kuhl (1999). *The Scientist in the Crib: What Early Learning Tells Us About the Mind*. Harper.

59. L. Murray (2014). *The Psychology of Babies: How Relationships Support Development from Birth to Two*. Robinson.

60. Ibid.

61. S. Pinker (2009). *Language Learnability and Language Development*. Harvard University Press.

62. B. Mampe, A. D. Friederici, A. Christophe & K. Wermke (2009). Newborns' Cry Melody is Shaped by their Native Language. *Current Biology*, *19*(23), 1994–7.

63. E. Bergelson & D. Swingley (2012). At 6–9 Months, Human Infants Know the Meanings of Many Common Nouns. *Proceedings of the National Academy of Sciences*, *109*(9), 3253–8.

64. Gopnik, Meltzoff & Kuhl, 1999. T. Cameron-Faulkner (2017). Language Development in the Young Child. In S. Powell & K. Smith (Eds). (2017). *An Introduction to Early Childhood Studies* (91–102) (4th ed.). Sage.

65. S. J. Hespos & K. van Marle (2012). Physics for Infants: Characterizing the Origins of Knowledge about Objects, Substances, and Number. *Wiley Interdisciplinary Reviews: Cognitive Science, 3*(1), 19–27.

66. B. Pettitt (2015). *Bringing Five to Thrive Alive: Two Approaches to Implementing Five to Thrive Within Barnardo's.* Barnardo's.

67. G. Wall (2010). Mothers' Experiences with Intensive Parenting and Brain Development Discourse. *Women's Studies International Forum, 33*(3), 253–63.

68. S. Lawler (2000). *Mothering the Self: Mothers, Daughters, Subjects.* Routledge.

69. A. O'Reilly (2016). *Matricentric Feminism: Theory, Activism, Practice.* Demeter Press.

70. C. Faircloth (2023). Intensive Parenting and the Expansion of Parenting. In E. Lee, J. Bristow, C. Faircloth & J. Macvarish. *Parenting Culture Studies* (33–67) (2nd ed.). Palgrave Macmillan.

71. C. E. Bolch, P. G. Davis, M. P. Umstad & J. R. Fisher (2012). Multiple Birth Families with Children with Special Needs: A Qualitative Investigation of Mothers' Experiences. *Twin Research and Human Genetics, 15*(4), 503–15.

72. A. Frederick (2017). Risky Mothers and the Normalcy Project: Women with Disabilities Negotiate Scientific Motherhood. *Gender & Society, 31*(1), 74–95.

73. Turmel, 2008.

74. Gopnik, 2016.

Conclusion: Embracing Motherdom

1. L. Jones (2023). *Matrescence: On the Metamorphosis of Pregnancy, Childbirth and Motherhood.* Penguin Books.

2. D. Levy (2018). *The Cost of Living: Living Autobiography 2.* Penguin Books.

3. A. Rich (1986). *Of Woman Born: Motherhood as Experience and Institution* (2nd ed.). W. W. Norton & Company.

4. A. P. Gumbs (2016). Introduction. In A. P. Gumbs, C. Martens & M. Williams (Eds). *Revolutionary Mothering: Love on the Front Lines* (109–10). Between the Lines.

5. J. C. Nash (2018). The Political Life of Black Motherhood. *Feminist Studies, 44*(3), 699–712.

6. R. Rapoport, R. N. Rapoport & Z. Strelitz (1977). *Fathers, Mothers, and Others: Towards New Alliances*. Routledge & Kegan Paul.

7. A. Garbes (2022). *Essential Labor: Mothering as Social Change*. Harper Wave.

8. R. Shah (2022). Losing My Mother Tongue: India and England. In C. Hull, R. Shah, C. Solomon, et al. *Our Mothers Ourselves: Six Women from Across the World Tell Their Mothers' Stories* (37–59). Austin Macauley.

9. A. O'Reilly (2016). *Matricentric Feminism: Theory, Activism, Practice*. Demeter Press.

10. Z. Sharman (2021, 21 April). With Queer Co-Parenting, the More is Definitely the Merrier. *Xtra*.

11. P. Agarwal (2021). *(M)otherhood: On the Choices of Being a Woman*. Canongate Books.

12. Interview with Robert Karen quoted in R. Karen (1994). *Becoming Attached: First Relationships and How They Shape Our Capacity to Love*. Oxford University Press.

13. C. Hardyment (2007). *Dream Babies: Childcare Advice from John Locke to Gina Ford* (2nd ed.). Frances Lincoln.

14. J. Randles (2021). 'Willing to Do Anything for My Kids': Inventive Mothering, Diapers, and the Inequalities of Carework. *American Sociological Review*, 86(1), 35–59.

15. P. Fielding-Singh (2021). *How the Other Half Eats: The Untold Story of Food and Inequality in America*. Little, Brown Spark.

16. E. Ross (1993). *Love and Toil: Motherhood in Outcast London, 1870–1918*. Oxford University Press.

17. K. Jeske (2014). It Could Be So Different: Truth-Telling, Adoption, and Possibility. In M. F. Gibson (Ed.). *Queering Motherhood: Narrative and Theoretical Perspectives* (159–68). Demeter Press.

18. A. Lorde (2007). *Sister Outsider: Essays and Speeches*. Crossing Press.

19. J. Clements & K. Nixon (2022). *Optimal Motherhood and Other Lies Facebook Told Us: Assembling the Networked Ethos of Contemporary Maternity Advice*. MIT Press.

20. A. Kamenetz (2020, 27 July). I Was a Screen-Time Expert. Then the Coronavirus Happened. *New York Times*.

21. R. Solnit (2017). *The Mother of All Questions: Further Feminisms*. Granta Books.

22. T. Miller (2024). *Motherhood: Contemporary Transitions and Generational Change*. Cambridge University Press.

23. R. H. Keefe, C. Brownstein-Evans & R. S. Rouland Polmanteer (2016). Having Our Say: African-American and Latina Mothers Provide

Recommendations to Health and Mental Health Providers Working with New Mothers Living with Postpartum Depression. *Social Work in Mental Health*, 14(5), 497–508.

24. S. Knott (2019). *Mother: An Unconventional History*. Penguin.

25. R. Parker (2005). *Torn in Two: The Experience of Maternal Ambivalence* (2nd ed.). Virago.

26. B. Almond (2010). *The Monster Within: The Hidden Side of Motherhood*. University of California Press.

27. E. Homewood, A. Tweed, M. Cree & J. Crossley (2009). Becoming Occluded: The Transition to Motherhood of Women with Postnatal Depression. *Qualitative Research in Psychology*, 6(4), 313–29.

28. Quoted in M. Benn (2006, 28 October). Deep Maternal Alienation. *Guardian*.

29. H. Lerner (1998). *The Mother Dance: How Children Change Your Life*. HarperCollins.

30. J. Raphael-Leff (2001). *Pregnancy: The Inside Story* (2nd ed.). Karnac Books.

31. L. Segal (2023). *Lean on Me: A Politics of Radical Care*. Verso.

32. T. F. Charlton (2013). The Impossibility of the Good Black Mother. In A. N. Nathman (Ed.). *The Good Mother Myth: Redefining Motherhood to Fit Reality* (177–84). Seal Press.

33. C. N. Adichie (2017). *Dear Ijeawele, or a Feminist Manifesto in Fifteen Suggestions*. 4th Estate.

34. A. Gopnik (2016). *The Gardener and the Carpenter: What the New Science of Child Development Tells Us About the Relationship Between Parents and Children*. The Bodley Head.

35. b. hooks (1984). *Feminist Theory: From Margin to Center*. South End Press.

36. O'Reilly, 2016.

37. M. Wollstonecraft (1792). *A Vindication of the Rights of Woman: With Strictures on Political and Moral Subjects*. The Project Gutenberg.

38. N. Scheper-Hughes (1992). *Death Without Weeping: The Violence of Everyday Life in Brazil*. University of California Press.

39. S. De Beauvoir (2015). *The Second Sex*. Translated by C. Borde & S. Malovany-Chevallier. Vintage Books.

40. D. V. M. Bishop (2018). Fallibility in Science: Responding to Errors in the Work of Oneself and Others. *Advances in Methods and Practices in Psychological Science*, 1(3), 432–8.

41. D. V. M. Bishop (2020). The Psychology of Experimental Psychologists: Overcoming Cognitive Constraints to Improve Research: The 47th Sir Frederic Bartlett Lecture. *Quarterly Journal of Experimental Psychology*, 73(1), 1–19.

42. R. L. Wasserstein & N. A. Lazar (2016). The ASA's Statement on p-Values: Context, Process, and Purpose. *The American Statistician, 70*(2), 129–33.

43. H. E. Longino (1990). *Science as Social Knowledge: Values and Objectivity in Scientific Inquiry.* Princeton University Press.

44. Full Fact (2020). *The Full Fact Report 2020: Fighting the Causes and Consequences of Bad Information.*

45. A. Cornwall & R. Jewkes (1995). What Is Participatory Research? *Social Science & Medicine, 41*(12), 1667–76.

46. World Vision/Ipsos (2023). *Not Enough: Global Perceptions on Child Hunger and Malnutrition.*

47. M. Kendall (2020). *Hood Feminism: Notes from the Women White Feminists Forgot.* Bloomsbury Publishing.

48. C. Humphreys, R. K. Thiara & A. Skamballis (2011). Readiness to Change: Mother–Child Relationship and Domestic Violence Intervention. *British Journal of Social Work, 41*(1), 166–84.

49. D. Roberts (2022). *Torn Apart: How the Child Welfare System Destroys Black Families – And How Abolition Can Build a Safer World.* Basic Books.

50. B. Featherstone, A. Gupta, K. Morris & S. White (2018). *Protecting Children: A Social Model.* Policy Press.

51. C. Collins (2019). *Making Motherhood Work: How Women Manage Careers and Caregiving.* Princeton University Press.

52. See M. Doepke & F. Zilibotti (2019). *Love, Money, and Parenting: How Economics Explains the Way We Raise Our Kids.* Princeton University Press. L. Scott (2020). *The Double X Economy: The Epic Potential of Empowering Women.* Faber & Faber.

53. B. Taggart, K. Sylva, E. Melhuish, et al. (2015). *Effective Pre-school, Primary and Secondary Education Project (EPPSE 3–16+): How Pre-school Influences Children and Young People's Attainment and Developmental Outcomes Over Time.* Department for Education. A. S. Bustamante, E. Dearing, H. D. Zachrisson & D. L. Vandell (2022). Adult Outcomes of Sustained High-Quality Early Child Care and Education: Do They Vary by Family Income? *Child Development, 93*(2), 502–23. D. L. Vandell, J. Belsky, M. Burchinal, et al. (2010). Do Effects of Early Child Care Extend to Age 15 Years? Results from the NICHD Study of Early Child Care and Youth Development. *Child Development, 81*(3), 737–56.

54. C. Criado Perez (2019). *Invisible Women: Exposing Data Bias in a World Designed for Men.* Chatto & Windus.

55. The Commission on a Gender-Equal Economy (2020). *Creating a Caring Economy: A Call to Action.* Women's Budget Group.

56. M. Marmot, J. Allen, T. Boyce, et al. (2020). *Health Equity in England: The Marmot Review 10 Years On*. Institute of Health Equity.

57. M. Zhavoronkova & R. Khattar (2021, 7 October). Investing in Home Care and Early Childhood Educators Has Outsize Impacts on Employment. *Center for American Progress*.

58. hooks, 1984.

59. D. Roberts (2017). *Killing the Black Body: Race, Reproduction, and the Meaning of Liberty* (2nd ed.). Vintage Books.

60. Dobbs v. Jackson Women's Health Organization, 19 US 1392 (2022).

61. S. B. Hrdy (1999). *Mother Nature: Maternal Instincts and How They Shape the Human Species*. Ballantine Books.

Index